D0982309

living with a man who is dying

living with a man who is dying

A PERSONAL MEMOIR

JOCELYN EVANS

New York | Taplinger Publishing Company

First published in the United States in 1971 by
TAPLINGER PUBLISHING CO., INC.
New York, New York

Library of Congress Catalog Card Number: 74-166177

ISBN 0-8008-4930-2

living with a man who is dying

1

We first met in perhaps the most conventional way, at a party thrown by a mutual friend. It was on a Saturday in late spring or early summer. I had been swimming and sunbathing most of the day, and sort of glowed with the additional energy that you get from direct contact with the sun. I don't remember the exact date, but Aron always claimed he fell in love with me the moment he saw me; years later he once mentioned that he still knew when it was.

I think I took a week or two to fall in love with him. My most vivid memory of the marvellous period that followed is of sitting on a bus with him, going to my flat. There was no way of getting close enough together on the bus, and it seemed that everybody around us must notice the extraordinary state of tension we were in. It was so obvious what would happen the moment we were alone together that just to look at him was like shouting it out all over the bus.

I never really expected anything like this to happen to me. For years I had imagined I was too unattractive. I suppose I stopped thinking that around the age of twenty when somebody I felt I hardly knew, and never would know well, immensely surprised me by proposing marriage. Then there were one or two young men who quite simply wanted to go to bed with me. But they weren't very difficult to resist. I had romantic ideas about what it should mean to go to bed with anyone. There had to be complete involvement at every level.

7

Liking and admiration had to be at least as strong as physical attraction. The love affair with Aron was particularly wonderful because it was the first time that all this was true.

It was so good, what there was between us, that actually getting married seemed a conceivable way of spoiling it. And certainly, considering the passion of that first summer, it took us an unfathomably long time to marry. We very nearly didn't. It's hard to remember now exactly what all the debating was about. I think it began with me developing the notion that marriage would put an end to some kind of independence I thought I valued. I worked this up to a pitch where we actually stopped seeing each other for a time. In fact, I nearly lost Aron because of some crazy idea I had about pursuing my career instead. He always respected my ideas, and he began to think along the same lines. In the end it was I who had to convince him that we should marry.

We were married in church—mainly because of me, because of the religious doubts to which I still half-heartedly clung; Aron was unaggressively agnostic. But we both thought it a splendid wedding. My parents organised it with such touching attention to detail, and the June sun shone all day. It was just over four years after we first met. We were both twenty-seven.

My background was Scottish, middle-class, academic. My father was a university professor, and my mother ran an infant school in Edinburgh from around the time that I went up to university. I had been brought up to take for granted most of the things that Aron had to earn with his brains.

This was an attraction to him, in the way that some of his working-class background was an attraction to me. There was a romantic aura attached to having working-class parents among left-wing university graduates of our generation. Admittedly Aron only just qualified as working-class. His father had risen, through sheer hard work, from the position of salesman to a desk in the Head Office of a large car company. But his grandfather (proud boast) had been a coalminer in the Rhondda Valley.

A thing that pleased me more than anything was the fact that this grandfather, whom I met only once, obviously liked me a lot. Physically he resembled Aron quite markedly. He had the same slim build, the same suggestion of asceticism, and I remember thinking how pleasant it showed Aron himself would be as an old man—gentle and inquiring and full of a quiet, independent kind of dignity.

Aron was an only son and an only grandson, the only nephew of several uncles and aunts. The whole family therefore watched him grow up with a particular love and pride. And he had always fulfilled their highest expectations. At school he was top of the class and good at sports, an excellent all-rounder. He went on to win an exhibition* to Oxford. For his grandfather, who had the pure, clean faith in education that you find especially among the Welsh and Scottish working-classes, this was a great day.

So, to a moving extent, was the day that Aron married me. I was well regarded by all his family. They liked the idea of my academic father, and the fact that I had my own career in journalism. They liked Aron's choice.

Of course we felt that we had grown rather far away from our family backgrounds by the time we got married. We were both much less conventional, or so we thought. We were certainly more cynical, mainly perhaps because neither of us had found the kind of work that satisfied our idea of what it was worth while to do in life. In spite of all his early promise, Aron got a clerical job with an insurance company and remained there, always frustrated and yet never able to find anything better or more right for him. We were both aware of a huge potential going to waste, and certainly we were bitter about it, and compensated for it perhaps by the depth of our relationship with each other. We had our own world, and there at least the priorities were sane.

At that time I was doing publicity writing in films, a job that I regarded as selling-out in the interests of doing any writing at all. Drop-outs weren't a feature of the 'fifties, and anyway

*A type of scholarship.

we were both too puritanical ever to have seriously considered dropping out. But we felt nonetheless trapped by the system. We opposed the kind of society that was content to waste, instead of making use of us. This is probably the main reason why we never got round to having children. We had somehow to justify our own existence first. It seemed wrong to have children in the hope that they would justify it for us.

I think that Aron really regarded most of his working life as a sham; reality was in the evenings and weekends, and on holiday. He never went anywhere without taking practically a whole suitcase full of books with him. On our honeymoon we lugged a small library on and off local trains and buses almost the entire length of the French Riviera. I read a good deal less than Aron, but I never doubted the need for this. I had always taken it for granted that where I went, lots of books went with me. They were a necessity of life, part of a constructive freedom of which Aron got too little. He didn't escape on holiday. He became himself. It seemed to me then that people who needed to have their spare time organised for them were the real escapists. I never saw Aron wondering what to do. Time was always against his doing half the things he wanted.

We usually went abroad for holidays, to Italy or Denmark if not France. But most often we went to Brittany. We would fly as far as Cherbourg or Dinard, and every time there was that feeling of absolute release the moment we set foot on foreign soil. The first Pernod sipped in blazing sunshine: there was always blazing sunshine on our holidays then. The first long, leisurely meal set out on a checked tablecloth. Nightfall in the old town of St. Malo, with its lighted café windows and Gallic bagpipers and historic ramparts overlooking the sea.

Then off along the coast to Sables-d'or-les-Pins, Erquy, Le Val André. Or south through thickly vegetated country to sleepy towns like Redon, where the chiming of the medieval church clock and the shunting of goods trains on the Paris-Bordeaux line nonetheless kept us awake all night. Travelling on in crowded local trains towards Quimper, peasant women in black clothing gave me disapproving stares—perhaps because my sleeveless dress exposed bare shoulders, I'm not sure. Yet Quimper was the place that had the most primitive public lavatory that I had ever seen, for the use of both sexes and awash with urine. It was refreshing somehow to find such different conventions being taken seriously. You could begin to regard your own traditional attitudes with a good deal more detachment and more humour.

In Quimper, the first time we got there, it was raining. We found the tabac where you waited for the bus to our ultimate destination, Beg-Meil. In Beg-Meil, they assured us, it would be fine. They were right. In Beg-Meil, in all our knowledge of the place, it was always fine. There was a view that you got between stone and trees, as you rounded the bend under the bridge on the road—a patch of bright sea and bobbing coloured boats, that at once proclaimed this as the special haven we had always looked for. Everywhere the scents were magnificent, but especially where the pine trees grew down to the sea's edge, mingling salt with resin. A great pine forest was said to have once stretched from here right across Brittany and all the intervening sea to Bournemouth, linking Britain with France.

We returned to Beg-Meil other years. We must have spent a total of at least twenty days there in all our life together. The word time has no meaning when I compare those twenty days with all the acres of waste time stretching before and after— time of which no account is ever taken, and which vanishes virtually without trace.

We stayed in one of those comfortable, friendly *pensions* where it was such an economy to be married, for every room contained a large soft double bed of the sort that the English have a reputation for not liking. Full board was unbelievably cheap there if you occupied one room and one bed. Breakfast (huge amounts of coffee with freshly baked bread and bowls of home-churned butter) was brought to our bedside at whatever time we wanted in the morning. We dressed in the lightest

11

clothes and set off in the sunshine on a ten-mile walk inland to Fuesnant to sample the local cider, or along the open sands to the isolated Pointe de Mousterlin overlooking a vast expanse of empty sea. On the way back we usually had a swim before rushing, starving, to the lunch table.

'Monsieur, Madame,' the French guests would say, nodding politely as we appeared, drunk with the sun and flushed with health.

'Monsieur, Madame'—it was somehow more splendid being married in France than anywhere else. It was a state known and recognised to be enormous fun.

There was a general siesta after the long, long lunch washed down with Aron's favourite Muscadet, and sometimes we went to bed then too. Afterwards, more swimming and sunbathing and hours of reading in the quiet coves among the rocks.

There seems now to have been something rather like childhood about those days of innocence and no responsibility. I know I was reminded very much of childhood when we took the boat across the bay to Concarneau: holidays in the West Highlands of Scotland when I was five; going to Mallaig in the rowing boat with the outboard engine and peering down through clear depths of water to the other world on the sea-bed; the gulls screeching and circling above the harbour as the fishing boats brought in their haul.

And the hours of reading were like childhood too. You could regard this as a time of self-indulgence, not quite real, infer that real experience had barely touched us. But this would be to ignore that what we felt and thought then was somehow at the core of our existence. It expressed our style, our attitude, the strong, sure things that would always be there.

Reading is itself something that takes place on innumerable levels. It matters what the world around is like when you are reading. 'There are, perhaps, no days in our childhood lived so fully as those that we believe to have been left unlived, days passed with a favourite book . . .' wrote Proust. 'If today we chance to turn over those books of another time, it is only as the sole calendars we have kept of the days that are fled, and in the hope of seeing reflected on their pages the abodes and pools that exist no more.'

So Mrs. Dalloway, pausing to look at Hatchard's window, is inextricably associated in my mind with the study-bedroom where I first read Virginia Woolf, and also with the warm sands of Finistère where Aron and I both read her again. Favourites on holiday were D. H. Lawrence and Thomas Mann, George Orwell and J. D. Salinger; Kingsley Amis because he made me laugh so much, though later I decided that he probably admired precisely what I most deplored; some poetry, Dylan Thomas for Aron, T. S. Eliot's *Four Quartets* for me.

After dinner darkness fell quickly. We usually watched the sun setting over the sea. Those seemed exceptional sunsets, profound and challenging, the colours shifting from moment to moment, a succession of ravishing variations on the theme of change. But perhaps they were no better than other sunsets that go on happening every evening on all the edges of the earth. The harmony that we felt then was not just in the sunsets; it was in ourselves.

*   *   *

Start here

The year that my story begins we had been married for six years. We decided to go to the Basque country instead of Brittany for our holiday in June. We flew to Paris to spend a night there before catching the sud-express to the Spanish border. It was to be a shorter French holiday than usual because we wanted to visit Wales and Scotland later in the summer. As it happened, it was to be different in other ways too— colder and wetter and somehow more acrid in flavour. This holiday had a kind of sadness about it that I shall never begin to understand.

We hardly ever booked hotel rooms in advance; in June it wasn't usually necessary then. But when we arrived in Paris this time everywhere was full. It was already rather late at

13

night, and as we trudged around the area of the Rue Jacob with our usual complement of heavy literature, I became fairly bad-tempered and tired.

'Why is it we can't walk along the street like other people without bumping into each other all the time?' said Aron, who of course carried the bulk of the load.

'Oh, I'm fed up with this,' I said, standing still and shouting. 'It's the middle of the night. Nobody else would expect me to walk about the streets looking for somewhere to sleep.' I knew of course that I was equally to blame for our situation. I was particularly reluctant to book in advance in case we changed our plans or disliked the hotels when we saw them.

Finally we found a place. It was both unattractive and expensive. There was broken glass in the washbasin, presumably what was left of the light bulb missing from the bedside lamp. We found we had forgotten to bring any soap. What that place charged for supplying a bar of soap made us thankful that we were leaving Paris in the morning. So it is that the wider view can be totally obscured by petty foreground details.

But the old French pleasure at being married had reasserted itself by the time we reached Bayonne. It was abroad that I was always most aware of the freedom that marriage gives and the status. All these things are relative. I suppose it's correspondingly worse to be a single woman in France. Actually I think there's no advantage in being a single woman anywhere I've ever been. By simply getting married, women still acquire a position in society that it's hard to equal in any other way.

Out in the career world only the exceptionally able and determined woman is likely to do anything other than play second-string, whereas there is equality in a good marriage. And of course, whether we acknowledge it or not, there are hundreds of little things that most women, even today, will hesitate to do on their own. I was accustomed to independence, to thinking I could do exactly what I liked. It even seemed possible beforehand that marriage might curtail this freedom. In fact it worked the opposite way. It wasn't just that there

14

was somebody to do things with. There was somebody to be independent and interested for.

In Bayonne it was always raining. For hours we sat and watched it from café terraces. We did a lot of walking, and we visited Biarritz a number of times. There, in the Maritime Museum, you lost all sense of place and time. You could have been gazing out of the past or out of the future at those congregations of prehistoric deep-sea fishes in their glass-sided pools. And the seals that lived on the roof—from what culture had they sprung? What strange inheritance had endowed them with their obvious liking for humans?

Once during a brief break of sunshine we bathed at Biarritz. We changed in a little canvas tent above the beach. In Britain we would have been directed to two separate tents, but there they automatically gave us the same one. There were cracks of sunlight coming through the joins of the green canvas. Aron took off his clothes. His body was beautiful. I was naked too, and suddenly almost dizzy with the kind of passion there had been between us the first time we made love so many years before.

The last of the little places that we visited was Bidart, the Basque equivalent of Beg-Meil, but slightly larger and not as pretty. Here it was impossible not to be aware of the hardships of life in a small fishing community, the strange green shrine to the madonna on the sea's edge, the cemetery practically adjoining one of the hotels. Aron who had recently become markedly averse to cemeteries, immediately rejected the possibility of staying in that particular hotel. But the cemetery was at the centre of the village and you passed it all the time. It looked as if somebody scrubbed and polished it regularly each day; it was in our opinion unhealthily well kept.

The weather continued in the main too cold and wet for sunbathing and swimming. We played miniature golf until we were quite good at it, and attempted long conversations in French in the hotel bar. Aron had developed a slight pain in his back, which sometimes prevented him from sleeping at night. He said once or twice that he thought he was ill, but I insisted on attributing the pain to the incessantly damp weather.

On our last day there we had a lengthy conversation with a middle-aged French couple who were at the beginning of a long and leisurely holiday. They had already been on holiday as long as we had, and they were now going off into the Alps for an indefinite period; two days stood between us and the big city, the rush hour, business as usual. If only we could have had the strength to break with it all, to set off independently for nowhere in particular with no special aim in mind! Never had I felt this impulse more strongly, but my whole life was made up of individual instances of resisting such impulses. I had long since passed the point, I thought, where irresponsibility of this kind stood the slightest chance of winning.

And so we took our last stroll along the promenade at Bidart. There was no sunset to speak of, only a curious, paralysing depression almost indistinguishable from fear, as darkness fell about us. What caused it, this terror that I felt? I was insupportably afraid. It's not part of my everyday philosophy to explain such things in the light of what happens afterwards. I expect to be able to explain them at the time. What did it mean *then*?

Of course the weather changed the moment we boarded the sud-express for Paris. The journey was stiflingly hot. I felt desperately sad, and also conscience-stricken. It was my fault that the holiday had lasted only ten days. This had been my decision, and it was wrong. But there was no way of reversing it now. My mood was like a continuation from the previous evening on the promenade, and immediately we set foot in Paris I started to cry. I went on crying most of the short time that we were there. I put on dark glasses, but I cried so much that everybody must have seen the tears streaming down my cheeks.

Aron accepted this extraordinary state of affairs as if it were quite normal. While we were strolling along the Quais, he even said that I looked wonderful. In the circumstances it was an incredibly nice thing to say, but it failed to make me control myself. What was it all about? Could we both have been aware, emotionally, intuitively, of something that neither of us actually knew until much later?

Back at home, life resumed its normal pattern for a time. We had recently bought a new flat, and had just about finished furnishing and equipping it. Aron had no enthusiasm for practical things. He hated shopping and do-it-yourself activities in particular. If a fuse had to be mended or a nail hammered into anything, I did it. On the other hand, he often cooked our supper and at weekends he nearly always brought me tea in bed.

By this time I had found a much more suitable job as a part-time editorial assistant on a literary magazine. I wrote film reviews for it, and Aron contributed occasional book reviews. It gave him an outlet for self-expression that his own job lacked, and he was also very involved in my writing. You usually get astonishingly little reaction to anything you write, and I relied substantially on his support and interest in what I was doing. I remember thinking, as I walked home one ordinary afternoon that summer, that life just went on getting better all the time now. Six years of marriage had shown that Aron and I had far more in common than we'd ever realised at first. Sometimes it seemed as if he knew more clearly than I did, how my mind worked.

At the August bank holiday we spent a few days with his parents in Wales. He was still suffering from the pain in his back that seemed to have begun in France. He had gone to the doctor about it, and X-rays had been taken. He heard the result of this the day we left for Wales. We travelled on the Pullman, facing each other across a little table. Aron looked tremendously well—slim and suntanned and sort of golden.

'I may be having an operation,' he said rather gently. 'There seems to be something the matter with my right kidney.'

He was smiling as he spoke. I smiled too, probably for the same reason, in an attempt to cover up concern. I remember it so clearly, with its sudden stab of fear, that sunny, smiling moment on the train to Wales.

Near the end of the journey the train passed very near the place where Aron had been born. It had changed a good deal, his birthplace, in the intervening years. Huge, dramatic slag-hills and perpetually smouldering furnaces now disfigured what had once been a very beautiful coastline. This was the first time I had seen it, because Aron's parents had only recently moved back to the area. I was interested and excited, more so I think than Aron who remembered very little of his childhood and always seemed reluctant to try to conjure it up. He felt, I think, some kind of guilt about his parents because they were content not to have had his opportunities in life. This is hard to formulate. Aron never formulated it himself, but it always seemed to me that he wanted his parents to want more for themselves. He sometimes mentioned how intelligent his father was, but how he never had the time or energy left to read the books that in fact interested him. Once he said of his mother, 'It's so sad to have been able to afford only one child!'

I have no idea why Aron was an only child. His parents were never really poor. On the other hand they always worked out what they could afford on an extremely realistic basis. Their lives never overflowed unpredictably in any direction. Whatever the circumstances and whoever was paying, for instance, tea in the best hotel in the district was regarded by Aron's mother as rather too great a luxury to be indulged in. So were taxis on most occasions for herself and her husband, although it became accepted that Aron and I were people who travelled in them when we wanted. It wasn't meanness and it wasn't necessity; it was a kind of caution that had turned into a way of life.

Physically I could see Aron in each of his parents. The father had much the same build and shape of face, and the mother sometimes wore Aron's expression about the eyes. But she was a small, very matter-of-fact person who talked in general about shopping, cooking, practical matters. Aron had depths that seemed not to have been inherited from either parent, although the father was, I think, more aware than he pretended of things that neither of them were accustomed to putting into words. Obviously he had always needed to have more push and drive than Aron, but sometimes I wondered if Aron's education had, in a mysterious way, robbed him of those particular qualities. It was his education, I suppose, that made him regard what the world calls success with such conspicuous lack of enthusiasm.

When we arrived this time, Aron told his mother about the kidney trouble, and she said not to worry because it would be all right. She had had a stone removed from her kidney, and it was nothing to worry about. Only she couldn't eat food with a lot of fat in it, that was all. Aron had brought a large supply of pills with him, but still slept very badly because of the pain. Something about the whole set-up, Aron's physical discomfort, the possibility of an impending operation, induced a kind of claustrophobia in me. I felt irrationally possessive about Aron, wanted to be outside with him as much as possible, wished I was alone with him and far away elsewhere.

Aron's mother brought out some of the things that belonged to Aron, books that went back to his childhood, photographs of him in school cricket and football teams, the cricket sweater that he hadn't worn since he left Oxford. Would he take some of them away, so that she could get the place tidy? She was exceptionally tidy. Very few old objects were allowed to remain in her house. Not long before this she had disposed of all the furniture and bought a new lot. She was not a person who formed attachments to objects simply for their associations with the past.

There were, of course, things associated with Aron that she kept: snapshots of him as a baby and as a child in his first school cap. That weekend, probably for the first time, I formed a clear picture of his earliest years. As we sat on the beach where he once played, I could visualise the whole scene on that faraway day when he got coated with oil from some ship at sea, had to be scrubbed down and developed a rash that took months to clear up. But when the war came he went as an evacuee to live with his grandparents, and it was conceivably then that the umbilical cord attaching him to his mother finally snapped forever. Certainly she seemed to me always to think of him as the baby, the little boy, who was no more. I thought she hardly knew my Aron.

On our last day there it poured practically the whole time. We all took a bus to Mumbles pier, hoping that the rain would stop by the time we arrived there. If anything, it got heavier. We sheltered in the arcades, tried our luck with the fruit machines. Aron was silent and stoical as we waited for the bus back. The pain was obviously considerable. We grumbled about the weather, but it wasn't the weather that was spoiling this weekend.

When we left, Aron's mother pressed a note into his hand. 'For the taxi,' she said as he protested and tried to give it back. 'Just take it for the taxi.' This always happened every time we went away. It must have started when Aron first left home at seventeen to do his national service, and it was probably repeated at the beginning of every term when he went up to Oxford to live like a gentleman. It seemed wrong really. We indulged ourselves so much by comparison with them.

Not long after this my grandfather died. I went up to Scotland alone for the funeral. The only other time that we had spent a night apart since we married was when Aron went to his grandfather's funeral in Wales. It was Aron's family who decided that I shouldn't be there. They said the occasion wasn't suitable for me. I think this stemmed partly from an old-fashioned attitude that funerals were primarily male affairs, and partly from the class-consciousness of the middle genera-tion, who saw their working-class origins in a much less romantic light that I did. Aron didn't come to my grandfather's funeral ostensibly because work was piling up at the office, but really I think because he felt unfit to travel.

My grandfather was cremated. It was the first time that I had been to a cremation. It gave me no sense of actually experiencing anything. I didn't see the body, or even feel particularly conscious of death. Anything that might have triggered off a sense of the reality of what had happened was covered up, kept out of sight. It reminded me of church services as a child, when all the children trooped into the vestry for Sunday school as soon as the main sermon began. I supposed that, during the main sermon, the adults got to grips with whatever it was that transformed the Bible stories from fairy tales into reality. But the more I participated in peculiarly adult activities, the less likelihood there seemed of ever receiving this kind of initiation. At my first communion I was still hoping that the things I was pretending to believe would suddenly become the things that I believed. For years I remained a member of the church, always arguing with myself as to whether or not it was hypocrisy to eat the bread and drink the wine and still feel absolutely nothing. This cremation was the same kind of thing. We had assembled together because of something that we never in any way confronted. How was it possible to make so little of the colossal, mysterious fact of death?

Aron had arranged to meet me at the railway station when I got back. All the way I was looking forward to the moment of being with him again, of dropping into that easy communication of ours that embraced so much and went so deep.

I saw him standing behind the barrier as I walked along the platform. He was wearing a blazer and an open-necked green shirt, and his mop of red-gold hair had reached the attractive length that his mother would have called too long. But he looked listless, withdrawn, and the way he greeted me was almost casual.

'What's wrong?' I said, disappointed at not having received the huge hug that I anticipated.

'Oh, nothing. Let's just get home.'

'Have you managed all right? Did you have enough to eat?'

'Yes, I wasn't very hungry.'

'Aren't you glad to see me?'

'Of course I am,' he said, as if I should have taken it for granted. 'I'm just tired.'

'I think you can't look after yourself,' I said. 'Or is it railway station Angst?' This condition, as analysed by Cyril Connolly in Aron's favourite, *The Unquiet Grave*, was something from which he claimed to suffer acutely. He smiled then, and quickly turned and led me away through the crowds.

2

The next event of any significance that I remember was Aron's examination at a central teaching hospital by a consultant to whom he had been referred by our G.P. I got home before he did, because he had conscientiously gone into the office after he left the hospital. He finally arrived looking very tired indeed.

The examination had apparently been conducted by a number of doctors, and was extremely thorough. They had asked him a great many questions about his appetite, his weight, the colour of his skin: was he sun-tanned or was he yellower than usual? However, he said that before he could tell me any more about it, he would have to go to the doctor and get a prescription. Otherwise the surgery*hour would be over. I was angry that he hadn't got a prescription at the hospital. 'Didn't they offer you something for the pain?' I said. Apparently nobody had thought about it. The subject hadn't come up.

This was Monday, and Aron hadn't had any pills all weekend. He had gone for a prescription on Saturday morning but there was nobody at the doctor's house, and a notice on the door informed patients that, due to the illness of one of the partners, the usual surgery was cancelled. Later he tried to ring the doctor about it, but calls were being referred to a telephone answering service which apparently had no method of dealing with matters of such minor urgency. It was a fifteen-minute

*Doctor's office.

23

walk to the doctor's, and there was no bus that went that way. On Saturday I had got the impression that it was almost too much for Aron. Walking was beginning to tire him out. I said I would go instead this time. I could easily collect the prescription for him.

At the weekend it had occurred to us that we should perhaps change our doctor. I knew that this was a comparatively simple matter under the National Health Service, because I had once done it when I was living in another town and had experienced similar difficulty in contacting the doctor who was supposed to be treating me. I think we decided against it this time because of all that had happened already, because of the X-rays that had been taken and the apparent liaison with the consultant. It would certainly have seemed likely to confuse things had we found another doctor at this stage.

When I arrived at Dr. Stella Sciberas' large, imposing residence, the part of it set aside for patients was teeming with people. But the doctor herself wasn't there. She finally made her appearance nearly an hour after the time that surgery was due to begin, practically the time it usually ended, so that it was understandable that she should want to rush people through. This she did with a vengeance.

'Want a certificate?' she said to me, before I had time to tell her that I had come about my husband and not myself. It was the first time that I had met her, although Aron had registered us both with her some time before. I needed to feel terribly ill to go near a doctor on my own behalf. I explained that I had come about my husband.

'Does he want a certificate?' she said, her pen poised ready to sign the thing at once. Noting my uncomprehending expression, she added, 'Does he want to stay away from work?'

I had no idea how to answer this question, and her obvious impatience was making me feel nervous.

'Do you know about him?' I said. She was a large woman of about fifty, with strong features and dyed blonde hair pulled back into a fairly sophisticated bun. She wore a costume of grey suiting and an impeccably fresh, frilled blouse. I felt extremely conscious of wasting her time, and that of everybody else in the waiting room, by not coming to a quick decision about the certificate.

'What's his trouble?' she said, her pen still poised, her expression far from solicitous.

'Well,' I said, 'he has a pain which I think is in his kidney. He was examined at the Northcote today, and I think he's going to have a barium meal X-ray.'

Dr. Sciberas got up and started to pace about beside the open door of the room. There were other patients just outside in the corridor, and I got the uncomfortable feeling that the interview was being conducted virtually in public.

'A barium meal?' she said. 'That's not for the kidney.'

I didn't take in her further description of the anatomical position of the kidneys in relation to the other organs. I was too alarmed. She had presumably one of these very literal minds that made her see it as a duty to correct me on my facts. But in my total ignorance of anatomy and medicine, the only fact that I grasped was that the illness was other than we had had been told. This was terrifying.

'Do you know about him?' I said again.

'No. My partner must have seen him. Do you want this certificate?'

'Yes,' I said. Aron had seen Dr. Sciberas at least once recently, but presumably she had forgotten. 'I don't know really whether he should go to work or not. I came for something for the pain.'

'The pain,' she said, writing as fast as she could now.

'The previous lot of pills only lasted a few days,' I said. 'And when he came here on Saturday, there wasn't a surgery.'

'My partner, Dr. Sidebotham, was ill.' She handed me the certificate and a prescription together. 'This will last a fortnight,' she said with a quick smile.

I went to the nearest chemist, a tiny place like a kiosk, which had remained open to cater for the people coming out of this surgery. It was dispensing huge quantities of mainly small white tablets to an endless line of weary-looking people. There seemed to be so few small white tablets in my bottle that I counted them before I left. If taken as directed, they would last only a week. I told the chemist what Dr. Sciberas had said, at which he became extremely angry.

'It's difficult enough to read her writing at the best of times,' he shouted, as if it were my fault. 'But that's what it says on the prescription.'

I had to go back to Aron and not let him see how desperately worried I now was. We had close friends, Dylan and Irma Jones, who lived in one of the streets that I passed on my way back. I thought of dropping in and telling them about it. But how could I do that? How could I tell them something that I wasn't going to tell Aron? It was impossible.

I think that Aron was really feeling too ill to notice my anxiety. He had an awful night. He paced about the flat in pain, and finally began to vomit. I lay there stiff with worry, deciding that in the morning I would have to ring the consultant. Did he know how bad the pain was? Aron probably hadn't told him. Did he anticipate the vomiting? I imagined that speaking to him would solve something, although I considered it a drastic method.

I hated all contacts with the medical profession. I think I had been afraid of doctors since one of them thrust a spoon down my throat at the age of two. I had an illness then which I now believe to have been largely psychosomatic and probably induced by my feelings about the birth of my brother. The rage and indignity that I felt about that spoon were out of all proportion to the event itself. A kind of anger was triggered off that never quite subsided. It remains I think at the heart of all my anti-authoritarian attitudes, my hatred of systems, of the establishment, of everyone and everything that thinks it has the right to thrust things down my throat without my prior permission.

But I suppose that in the end I really rang the consultant

for reassurance. I regretted it later as the act of panic it had been. I shouldn't have interfered. I should have let things take their natural course.

When the consultant heard about the pain and vomiting, or when he heard me obviously panicking perhaps, he decided to admit Aron to hospital at once. I was relieved, temporarily. I thought that somebody else had taken over the responsibility. I had still to learn that it isn't as simple as that. Responsibilities can never really be taken over by anybody else.

Aron wasn't relieved.

'They're taking you in,' I announced smilingly, as if he'd like the news.

'Oh,' he said, looking very miserable indeed. He was still in bed. Then he quietly got dressed, and went and sat down in the living room.

It was mid-September now, and ironically an Indian summer had just begun. Waiting for the ambulance to come, Aron sat in streaming sunshine beside the window, and said:

'I wish I was dead.'

Then he added, and this somehow frightened me far more: 'Why do I feel so cold?'

Almost immediately pulling himself together, he suggested that I should sit outside and get some sun while I had the chance. I couldn't. The absurd reason was that I had too much of a pain in my stomach to relax at all. While I was packing one or two things into a bag for him, I had been practically doubled up with pain. I knew it was just nerves, just foolishness, but codeine had no effect on it. When the ambulance driver arrived, he looked from one to the other of us and said:

'Which of you is the patient?'

I liked the ambulance, all cool and shaded and organised inside. But Aron looked out at the empty street, its occupants all away at work, and said:

'It's as quiet as death!'

I wished he would stop mentioning death. I wished he wouldn't talk this way. These days too he was always saying how old he felt, or ill. Yet he was only thirty-three. He seemed to have an increasing reluctance to make any kind of physical effort. He used to sit and watch me gardening, for instance. Once, when I was transplanting the forget-me-nots in the hope that they would cover all the plots the following year, he said he wished he could do what I was doing.

'You move and bend so easily,' he said. 'You're so agile.'

'So are you, if you want to be,' I said.

'No. Not any more. I'm old and stiff. My life is practically over.'

I could make nothing of this kind of remark, and usually treated it rather impatiently. But there was something wrong. Aron hardly ever had the energy to make love now. More than once I suggested that his feelings towards me had changed.

'No,' he protested. 'I love you. You must believe I love you.'

I did believe it, but I was still sorry for myself. I had a lot to learn about what loving really means. As we drove away in the ambulance, my thoughts were really quite selfish. I wanted Aron to go to hospital and be made physically fit again for my sake. I wanted him to come back strong because of me.

*　　*　　*

The Northcote Hospital was a comparatively modern building with no particular character at all. It stood on a busy main road and, being a teaching hospital, was run with a reasonable amount of anonymous efficiency. Its narrow hallway, with blank cream walls and long padded benches for waiting people, would in my opinion have served very well as a model for the vestibule of hell in a novel by Franz Kafka. But as we walked through it, Aron suddenly looked at me and smiled like his old self. It was a smile so golden that I can believe it might still be shedding some light and personality about the place.

Then they led him off into an ante-room to undress. I saw him for only a second more, when I was given his clothes to take home. In his pyjamas and dressing gown he looked ill, and also apprehensive. But they didn't want me in the ward then. They said I could come back and see him in the evening, at visiting time. That was really when I first realised what a separation his being in hospital would mean. I hadn't thought of it that way till then.

Blinking back tears, I drifted out of the place alone, with no notion of what to do next. The only thing really was to take his clothes home. As I was hanging them up in the wardrobe I began to cry. I cried and cried then out of sheer loneliness. There had been so very few nights without him, and then I had always known exactly when we would be together again. This was miserable, not to know, and only to be able to see him at hospital visiting times. I think I had actually forgotten about my job at that point. I lost interest in it completely from the moment that Aron went into hospital.

That night I phoned Aron's parents and told them where he was. The news was hardly unexpected, and they took it quite calmly.

'You must be feeling lonely then,' said Aron's mother. Her Welsh accent (much stronger than her husband's, and not shared by Aron at all) gave all the words equal value until the end of each sentence when her voice rose to a small crescendo. 'You have hardly ever been separated, have you?'

The hospital tolerated visitors for half an hour each evening, and an hour on Thursday, Saturday and Sunday afternoons. At visiting times everybody waited in the entrance hall until the porter got the signal to let the throng surge past him along the various corridors and staircases towards the wards.

It depended on the individual sister whether or not you got straight into the ward you were visiting. At Aron's ward you always had to wait again outside the door. You stood there savouring what I think of as hospital smell—like a mixture of rubber, cooked cabbage and anaesthetics—while frantic, last-minute tidying went on behind the closed door. Sometimes you had to wait for as long as ten minutes, but I hardly ever heard anyone complain about it. Most of the other visitors had the air of habitués, and simply accepted this delay as part of the natural order of things. I certainly had no such attitude. But, like the others, I wouldn't have dared to complain about anything in case my patient suffered as a result.

Waiting outside the ward my anxiety about Aron always reached a kind of fever pitch, which I feared would reflect on the conversation we had when I finally got in. I felt so sorry for him, alone and worried, in the ward, and for myself, I suppose, alone and worried, outside it. Admittedly Aron read a lot, and as long as he had the books he wanted he could spend most of his time in a world of his own. But I was probably right in thinking he was lonely. It was a very busy surgical ward with over thirty beds in it, and nobody there had much in common with Aron except the young house surgeon, who had become a friend, but who had very little time.

Anyway, whether or not Aron needed me, I needed him. I really found it impossible to compress all that I needed of his company into half an hour. Time with him had seemed limitless till then. It embraced the whole present, coloured all the past and stretched far into the future making even old age an acceptable and pleasant prospect. For the first time I fully realised the extent of the happiness that I mostly took for granted.

When you got into the ward, all the nurses seemed to vanish and nobody came to meet you. Most of the patients were considerably older than Aron, and some of them looked frighteningly ill. I remember, the first time, the embarrassment of having to find Aron. I hardly dared look around too much for fear of what I might see. It seemed like an intrusion to be paying attention to the other patients at all. It was such a relief when Aron, sitting propped up against his pillows, saw me and beckoned me over to his bedside.

The bed next to Aron's nearly always had the curtains drawn around it.

'Poor chap!' Aron once whispered glumly. 'He's having a

rotten time.' He was an elderly man who had, apparently, had several operations, and who existed in a constant state of pain and discomfort. It seemed that he had no particular desire to live. Aron had heard him pleading with the nurses to leave him alone and let him die.

'What do they say to that?' I asked.

'They tell him not to be silly. They treat him like a child really.'

I still had virtually no idea what was wrong with Aron. Nobody at the hospital had approached me, and I didn't approach them. I don't know why. I got any news there was now from Aron himself. Nothing much seemed to be happening. He had still to have the barium meal X-ray, because the appointment for it was postponed when he became an in-patient instead of an out-patient. It looked as if the diagnosis depended on the result of this, and we were sorry that his admission to hospital had delayed it. We tried to talk about other things, but we kept coming back to that.

To announce the end of visiting times, two young patients (I suppose they were in their early teens, but they looked as if they ought to qualify for a children's ward) used to tear up and down the ward, ringing a hand bell for all they were worth. Any nurses who were around seemed to find this quite amusing. I found it disproportionately intolerable. I could hardly stand the noise, and neither I felt could some of the sick people for whom the place was supposed to be catering. Yet I took it for granted that it couldn't be stopped. Visit after visit, I suffered it in silence.

On the day that Aron should have had his barium meal X-ray, he was given food in error in the morning. As a consequence the X-ray had to be postponed for another four or five days. The purgatory of waiting was prolonged.

The jaundiced condition noticeable in the whites of his eyes just after he was admitted to hospital had worsened, then subsided. It was suggested that he might go home for the weekend, but the jaundice flared up again. After a dizzy turn in the washroom, he was told to stay in bed. Still, the weekend visiting hours were longer. There was time for me to try to encourage him to eat. He was hardly eating anything now, and the nurses were usually too busy feeding helpless patients to give the matter much attention.

When Aron finally had his barium meal X-ray, I thought it better to wait until the next day to inquire about it. I rang the consultant, Mr. Warfield-Scrogge*, before setting out for the office in the morning. His secretary said he wanted a personal word with me.

'We shall have to have a talk,' he said. 'But I don't really like discussing patients on the telephone.'

'Shall I come and see you?'

'Well, not today.' There was a pause. 'I am going to operate on your husband's stomach tomorrow,' he said. 'The operation will be of an exploratory nature.'

'Do you think . . . is it, is it serious?' I stammered.

'Yes,' he said after a moment. 'Yes, I'm afraid it is.'

'When can I see you?' My voice had become almost angry with fear.

'Come on Thursday afternoon,' he said, 'at visiting time.'

That was the day after tomorrow. Why did he want to wait until the day after tomorrow?

'He'll be all right? I mean, the operation will be all right?' I said.

'I can't be certain,' was his reply.

What was he saying? Was it as bad as I thought? I would be seeing Aron in the evening. What would I say to him?

'What does he know about this?' I said.

'I have told him that the operation is for the removal of a cyst,' said Mr. Warfield-Scrogge.

I spent the rest of the day nearly demented with fright. But I remembered that Aron had said he might phone me later in the morning in the office, so I went there in case he did. In the office they accepted that I was no longer any use. They watched me come and go without actually expecting me to

*British surgeons are addressed as Mr. rather than Dr.

accomplish anything. I think they probably preferred it when I didn't come at all.

Aron did in fact phone. He sounded unperturbed. I was so glad to hear him, especially somehow in the office. It was one of the normal things that happened, Aron phoning in the office. It was stability. For a moment or two the terror at the back of my mind seemed by comparison an unsubstantial thing.

Aron said that the operation would be on Thursday. How was that, I wondered? Was it really what he had been told, or was he trying to make the evening visiting time easier for me by concealing the fact that the operation was tomorrow? I kept forgetting that he had no idea how anxious I was. In fact, the operation was on Thursday.

I had lunch with Dylan, who had been a friend of Aron's since they were at Oxford together. While I think he felt that my fears about Aron must be exaggerated, he was concerned about the state I was in. He and Irma decided to move into my spare room that night. It was almost necessary as far as I was concerned. I wasn't coping any more. I let them organise everything. Irma went to see Dr. Sciberas, whom she had recommended to us and with whom she seemed to have an excellent relationship, and brought back a sedative for me. She also accompanied me to the hospital on the last visit before Aron's operation.

I was very afraid of being unable to carry off this occasion without breaking down completely. But as I approached the hospital I noticed that, almost despite myself, I was becoming calmer. Had I been religious, I would certainly have said that God was giving me strength. But of course I had strength anyway. I was very strong and healthy, and you might equally well argue that I had been making remarkably poor use of this in everything I had done, or failed to do, so far. Perhaps a little of my basic stamina was finally coming to the fore.

By now Aron was obviously alarmed. He kept running out of things to say, attempting to fill in silences that wouldn't at any other time have mattered. I couldn't help him. I was too certain that his fears were justified, too afraid myself. It was an impossible situation, but at least nobody broke down. And one good thing happened.

On the way out Irma put her feelings into action. She snatched the bell from the boy who was ringing it. 'That's quite enough,' she said. 'People who are ill don't like a noise like that.' Then she handed the offending thing to a nurse who stood vaguely smiling by the door. Apparently it only needed that kind of initiative to get it stopped. I never saw either of the boys with the bell again.

3

The morning of the operation came, bright and sunny like all the other mornings then. There was nothing to be done but stay beside the phone. I had no idea what time the operation would take place. I was even unsure that the hospital would ring me if things went badly wrong. There really had been practically no communication between me and anybody there so far. I blamed them for this, because I expected them to take the initiative. I expected them to appreciate that I was being considerate and not a nuisance. It never struck me that, because I wasn't constantly asking questions, they might be totally unaware of the extent of my anxiety. When a thing like this happens, it's hard to realise that other people may not think about you at all unless you draw their attention to your problems.

I was afraid to be alone. Jennie from the flat next door came in to keep me company while Irma was out teaching. Jennie was about twenty-one, blonde, pretty and expecting a baby. She talked solidly for about an hour and a half. She told me what everybody in the street was doing, what the new flats cost and how they were being decorated inside, what they said to her at the clinic, how she couldn't sleep just now but refused to take any drugs in case they harmed the baby. She was rather delightful company, and for moments on end succeeded in pushing the worry back a little. She had brought two huge pastries with her, which she insisted we had to eat. I made some coffee, and we were sitting drinking it in the living room when there was suddenly a huge noise, like thunder, in the hall.

We both leapt to our feet, quite at a loss to think what it could be. It was curious what had happened. Without any apparent reason—and certainly nobody was moving about in any of the flats because Jennie and I were the only people at home—the curved plasterboard cornice had fallen from the ceiling and broken into several pieces on the floor. Happening when it did, it was unnerving. I expected the phone call from the hospital any minute now. But no call came.

When Irma came back in time for lunch, there was still silence from the hospital. By now the operation must be over. I wonder why I didn't ring them up to find out what had happened. Was I afraid to ask? Of course, I have always been rather bad at asking. I have always felt that the more important the question, the more necessary it is to discover the answer for myself, to get the information first-hand. Perhaps it's a Scottish non-conformist trait to prefer, in general, to do things the hard way.

At last Irma was driving me to the hospital in time for the usual Thursday afternoon visiting hour at two o'clock. I had stopped seeing much of what went on around me. But occasionally isolated objects stuck out with peculiar clarity—unrelated images belonging to a world in which I wasn't really living. One particular Georgian house somehow imprinted itself on my memory as a result of one of these journeys. I could imagine leather-bound volumes in the library, piano music drifting across the lawn. Then a name above a shopfront showed we were nearing the hospital. Now none of the land-marks really mattered except as indications of the distance from that place. Getting nearer, worry blanked out everything between the street and the moment of reaching the ward.

Visitors were rushing past us on both sides. I didn't want to look for Aron until I had spoken to somebody about him. I found the sister* in her office.

'I'm Mr. Evans' wife,' I said.

*Head floor nurse in British hospital.

'Mr. Evans?' She rubbed her chin reflectively, as if the name conceivably could mean something to her. She was a compact little person, who might have been anything up to sixty years old. Small, greyish whiskers sprouted here and there from her face.

'Oh yes,' she said. 'We've moved him.' She motioned vaguely in a direction farther along the ward.

'Where?' I said hesitantly. Irma had tactfully hung back, and I couldn't understand why the sister didn't at least accompany me to Aron's bedside, why she seemed not to realise that this was what I wanted. Instead she took only a few steps out of her room and pointed again.

I started to walk diagonally across the ward to the far point under the window where Aron now lay. I felt impossibly conspicuous. I had to go through with this or everybody would see what a coward I actually was. Once, as an adolescent, I entered a diving competition without realising that it involved high diving. Plunging off the top board, which I had never even stood on before, was an experience just comparable to this.

Aron looked yellower and, at the same time, alarmingly waxen. He lay with his hands flat on the bedclothes at his sides, and his face set like an effigy. There were tubes coming out of his nose, and he was very still. It was a terrifying sight. Of course he was going to die.

When I spoke to him, he replied from a great distance.

'Awful . . . awful . . .' he seemed to be saying.

'I love you,' I said. 'I think of you all the time, all the time.'

I said it as if I were reciting a set speech. I was actually afraid of him. I was afraid of what he had become. I wanted to get away from him, to leave him to the people who had messed him up like this.

'I'll go now,' I said. 'But I'll come back.'

I turned away, clutching my head like an actor giving a very ham performance, and a coloured nurse came up quickly and took me by the arm.

'Come Mrs. Evans, dear,' she said. And looking into her

black, bespectacled face, I recognised real sympathy. Aron had mentioned her. She must be the nurse from Trinidad, the one who seemed genuinely to care.

She led me to the sister's office, where I made an exhibition of myself. Irma sat holding me while I moaned and groaned, and the sister tried to make contact with Mr. Warfield-Scrogge on the internal telephone. This state of affairs seemed to go on and on. Eventually the sister left us without apparently having contacted the surgeon. She came back with two brandies, which she offered to Irma and me. Irma said I had had a phenobarbitone (so that was what my pills were!) and that she was driving. The sister took the two brandies away. After another seemingly infinite period of time, which was probably about ten minutes, we were summoned into the presence.

We were being led through corridors and still more corridors. Shock had possibly affected my sense of perspective in space as well as time. I got the impression that the nurses guiding us changed over at intervals, as if the journey were too long for any one of them to act as escort the whole way. Latterly we seemed to be penetrating inner, narrower passages where guard nurses, stationed at strategic points, permitted entry only after muttered passwords had been exchanged. We were finally told to sit down, one behind the other, on tubular metal chairs immediately outside the surgeon's room. In a few moments the door opened.

Mr. Warfield-Scrogge rose to his feet from where he was sitting behind a desk in the small, ugly brown room. He was a tall, thin-faced man with unblinking, impersonal eyes.

'Mrs. Evans?' he said, glancing from one of us to the other. It was, of course, the first time we had met. I shook hands with him.

'This is my friend, Mrs. Jones,' I said. And he shook hands with Irma.

'Should I stay here just now?' she asked.

'Yes, I'd be glad if you would,' the surgeon said. 'I'd like somebody else to be here.'

He directed me to the chair opposite him, and Irma to the only other available chair which was against the wall.

'There is nothing I can do for Mr. Evans,' he said at once. 'There is absolutely no hope for him, and I think it will probably all be over very soon.'

I looked at the plain calendar on the wall behind him. It was the only thing to look at. The room was so bare that it was like a vacuum. I don't even remember a clock being there. This was, I supposed, as quick and clean an incision as the one that he had made into Aron's flesh earlier in the day. He was a man who used the knife with an assured technique. There was no indecision, no hesitation about anything he did.

He began on the details, which were intolerable. My mind battled to reject them, unsuccessfully. People have since assured me that the recipients of news like this can rarely remember with any accuracy what they have been told. I have no evidence of having forgotten very much of that hideous conversation. And certainly, things were said that day that nothing will ever erase from my memory. But I was obviously confused in many ways, and it is possible that, without realising it, I am now misquoting some of Mr. Warfield-Scrogge's remarks.

'You notice that he is rather yellow just now,' he said. 'Well, he will get yellower . . . perhaps ultimately greenish . . . But he won't suffer.'

'Not suffer?' I said.

'We can give him things that prevent it,' the surgeon replied rather gently. 'He will gradually drift away. By the end he probably won't know what's happening.'

'No,' I thought. 'No.' For Aron not to know what was happening to him seemed somehow worse than anything else.

'He will need you,' said Mr. Warfield-Scrogge. 'He will need you for as much of your time as you can possibly give him.'

I looked at him blankly. There was surely no relation between this and his previous remark. If Aron was barely conscious of anything that was happening, how could I possibly be of use to him? I hated the idea of Aron being deprived of his mental faculties. Even then, I hated that more than anything. I felt that whatever was happening, Aron would always prefer to be aware.

Perhaps the surgeon misinterpreted my expression, and thought that his remark about Aron needing me had made me feel too responsible. Apparently close relatives have a tendency to blame themselves for tragedies like this. Mr. Warfield-Scrogge may have thought that I was already blaming myself, because he went on to explain that the disease was due to something that had happened a long time ago, which nobody could have done anything to prevent.

But I wasn't blaming myself. I was the sort of person much more likely to blame the surgeon. I looked at his hands—long thin hands, inappropriately like those of an artist—the hands that had cut Aron open. And I suppose I hated them.

'Have you a family?' he said.

'Well, I have a mother and father . . .'

'No,' said Irma, understanding his question better. 'There aren't any children.'

'Do you want to ask me anything just now?' he said. 'Of course, you can come back and see me. You can see me any time.'

'What is it that he has?' I said.

'It's a cancer.'

'How long . . . how long is there?'

'I always think it wrong to answer that question. It's wrong of me to say. One shouldn't think in such precise terms . . . But I would put it at six weeks, or less.

'As time goes by, he may begin to realise. But he will never know. He must never know. We must never say anything that will kill hope. It's wrong to kill hope.

'For you,' he went on, 'the world will come to an end. There's no doubt of that. Everything will seem to be over. But later, gradually, you will find things beginning to take shape again. Life will start again . . . You are young. How do you feel? Will you be all right just now?'

40

'I'm not the sort of person likely to faint or anything, if that's what you mean,' I said. Then I mentioned that I had also had a phenobarbitone.

The smile that had been forming on his face, immediately vanished.

'A phenobarbitone! Why is that?'

'I got them for her from our doctor,' Irma explained.

'Who is your doctor?' he asked.

'Dr. Sciberas,' said Irma.

'Oh yes.' He appeared to know and approve of Dr. Sciberas. At least that's how Irma interpreted his tone of voice. Dr. Sciberas had never tried to communicate with me while Aron was in hospital. She never dropped in to see me, even after Irma told her how desperately worried I was. Also Aron and I had discussed our feelings about Dr. Sciberas during the ten days that he had been in hospital. We had decided that we would prefer a doctor who seemed to have more time to spare for patients. We intended to change our doctor as soon as this business was over. But there was no point in bringing this up with Mr. Warfield-Scrogge. Now it hardly mattered who our doctor was. At least it didn't matter to Aron, who would never be back home again.

'Stop taking the phenobarbitone,' said Mr. Warfield-Scrogge. 'Don't take any more.' I regarded this as healthy advice, and obeyed it implicitly. The phenobarbitone had had no noticeable effect anyway.

'Go home now,' he said, 'and come back and see your husband in the morning.'

'He expects me before then,' I said hesitantly.

'Why? Did you speak to him? What exactly did you say?'

'I said I'd come back.'

'Go home now, and come back tomorrow,' he repeated, as he knew I wanted him to do. He was ready to make my duty seem only as arduous as he thought me capable of performing.

So I left the hospital without going back to the ward where

Aron lay moaning, 'Awful . . . awful . . .' Had there been no opportunity to make up for it later, I doubt if I could ever have forgiven myself for this. I abandoned Aron on what he afterwards described as the worst day of his life.

*　　*　　*

The first thing I noticed when I got home was the gap where the cornice had been. When did it fall? Was it the moment when they looked inside him and saw death there? I've imagined the actual scene so often since. The surgeon and his assistants, hooded and swathed in green, bent over the huge raw cavity which is the only part of Aron not hidden by green towels. Only the eyes of the others are exposed above their masks, and the surgeon's piercing stare changes focus, blurs a little at what it sees.

'Looks like carcinoma. Head of the pancreas,' he pronounces. 'God, it's all over the place! Absolutely inoperable! Take a look.' And he stands aside to let the houseman see.

'He's only thirty-three years old,' a theatre nurse whispers in the wings. She is a white bundle in white tennis shoes, swaying towards a similarly clad figure beside her.

The surgeon demands an instrument with curt precision. Only a very perceptive observer could have noticed how, at that remark, he flinched. This is defeat. This is where being a surgeon differs from being God.

Aron, I decided must never know the cornice fell. Also he must be taken out of that ward. I rang Mr. Warfield-Scrogge, and asked for advice about moving Aron somewhere else. I thought he might become a private patient, or go into a nursing home. If this were only for six weeks, presumably we could afford whatever it cost. I had no idea what it would cost, or really what we could afford.

'It's absolutely out of the question for you to pay anything,' the surgeon said. 'And I can assure you that the treatment will be much better here than it would be in a nursing home. I'll have him moved to a side ward, with possibly one other patient. You will be able to visit him at any time there.'

I imagine that Mr. Warfield-Scrogge thought that my only objection to the ward was concerned with visiting. Obviously I could never have told him with what abhorrence I regarded it as a place in which to die.

*　　*　　*

The blackness and the faintness had gradually been replaced by glaring light and a roaring noise and pain. Pain again. Aron lay very still, and tried to concentrate on remembering what had happened.

'Oh God!' he thought. 'I'm alive. I'm still in the hospital. Why didn't I die?'

For a long time now, the easiest thing had really seemed to be to die. All his energy had somehow gone. What was he trying to remember? The pain was terrible. He couldn't be sure where it was. It just enveloped him. Was it pain, or was it something else? A huge part of him was bandaged. That must be where the pain was. And there was something sticking down his throat and out of his nose. Oh, awful!

A nurse was standing over him.

'You'll just feel a little prick,' she said.

'What . . . is . . . this?' he managed to say, dragging his hand up to the tube in his nose. His voice boomed strangely in his head.

'Just a little tube,' she said.

'Take it away.'

'I can't take it away yet. I'm sorry dear.'

Aron closed his eyes, drifted out a little, saw himself holding a huge beaker of thick, white liquid with a vanilla flavour. He had drunk so much of it that he felt stuffed right up to his neck.

'Now you can drink some more please,' said the radiologist. He had a mid-European accent. 'Try, do try.'

Aron gulped and gulped again. Some of it at least was going down.

'Good!' said the radiologist, who was watching the progress of the barium, from the stomach to the duodenum, on a small television screen on Aron's right.

'Now, don't move. Don't breathe. Keep still.'

There followed a succession of sharp clicks, as he shot a series of still photographs of the scene inside Aron's abdomen.

'Finish the beaker, right?'

Aron gulped hard. He was absolutely full. There was this tube too. That was the reason why he couldn't swallow. They ought to have thought of that.

'Take it away.' The sound of his own voice jolted him back to the present.

A nurse was holding his hand.

'Don't upset yourself,' she said. 'We'll take it away as soon as we can, as soon as the doctor says.'

This is a trap. I'm trapped. I can't escape. He saw himself like Gulliver among the Lilliputians, with little threads tethering every part of him to the hard bed. Only they weren't threads; they were tubes that went inside him, and only doctors could get them out.

Now she is here, my wife, he thought. I know it without looking. I know the sound of her, the way the air moves round her. I can see her in the garden, so lucky, so young and supple, digging up those plants—what were they called again, those plants? She is frightened. What a mess! Why doesn't somebody help? She has gone. Why has she gone? Why doesn't somebody take the tube out?

Then he came, the surgeon. He was compassionate.

'Is the tube bothering you so much?' he said. 'All right, we can take it out now,' he told the sister.

'You will be feeling pretty bad at the moment,' he said. 'But we are going to try to make things pleasanter for you, because you need a lot of rest. We discovered at the operation that there is something wrong with your liver. It will take a long time to get better. Would you like to go into a little room by yourself, where you wife can visit you more often?'

'Oh yes,' said Aron.

'All right. We'll move you there before tomorrow. And if you have any other problems, you will tell me, won't you?'

'Yes,' said Aron. 'Yes.' And he sank into a less troubled sleep.

4

I find that I no longer remember any conversation in which I told Aron's parents the news. Perhaps somebody else did it for me. Perhaps my father phoned them, because he came to stay with me around that time. He was able to come and stay since he had by now retired from his university chair. I'm not sure precisely when he came. The only things I remember easily are those that directly concerned Aron.

We never told Aron that my father had come to stay with me, because we thought he would wonder why. On the face of it, there was no reason for wanting somebody in the flat. I wasn't normally the sort of person who minded being alone. The circumstances would have had to be rather extreme for a member of my family to come from Scotland and live with me, and Aron would wonder what the extremity was.

For a time I was rather obsessed about ensuring that he shouldn't discover this lie. It would be half-way towards discovering the bigger lie which we were all now obliged to live, but which seemed at the beginning so impossible to keep from him. Actually I thought that I would give the show away the moment I saw him.

When I arrived in the ward the morning after the operation, Aron's friend, the young house surgeon Dr. Lewis, came to meet me at the door.

'He's in rather a lot of pain at the moment,' he said quickly.

'I'm such a coward,' I said. 'Come with me.' And I think I held out my hand.

'Yes, of course.' He smiled reassuringly. 'He's doing very well. You'll find him much brighter than he was yesterday.'

Dr. Lewis led me to the little side room which Aron now occupied on his own. In fact, he never had to share it with anybody else. But because of Mr. Warfield-Scrogge's original remark about this, I feared for quite a long time that another patient might be moved in any day.

There were large windows all along one wall, and sunshine flooded the place. Outside you could even see a few trees. The atmosphere was altogether changed.

'A visitor for you,' said Dr. Lewis cheerfully, and left us together.

There were no tubes now, and Aron looked a lot better. He welcomed me quite normally, and I sat down beside him. But every few minutes he was gripped by a terrible spasm of pain. At first I thought that this pain was part of the way he was going to die. I regarded each stab as an intimation of death. I thought that there was nothing I could do, that the pain, like the death to come, was something that neither of us could fight. At least I thought this until I held his hand.

It was extraordinary how things altered then, how he suddenly became Aron again instead of a dying thing that only medical people could help. He was Aron, and of course I could help him. It sounds trite, however put, but the effect of simply holding his hand was marvellous. It was as if he had been floundering about alone, and I had given him an anchor. We both seemed to have gained a sort of security beyond the realms of possibility a moment before.

'Everyone's being very kind,' he said, looking almost happy.

And so began the most intense, most unforgettable period in all our knowledge of each other. How could I be afraid any more when I was as close to him as this? What we meant to each other now was surely quite out of the usual, quite the nearest to perfection that a relationship between two people could ever reach.

My mother came for the weekend that night. She was a good deal younger than my father. Always much prettier than I had ever been, she was also attractive because her interest in other people so obviously exceeded her interest in herself. Aron once said it would delight him were I to resemble her at the same age.

'It's going to be easy for him anyway,' I protested to her. 'I'm going to make it easy for him.'

'How?' she said quietly, regarding me with puzzled gentleness.

I don't know what I replied. I doubt if I had any idea *how*. I just knew, from what had happened that day, that I could help Aron. I knew that I was going to make all the difference in the world to the kind of death he had.

But I doubt if my determination looked very convincing when I wasn't with Aron. It was only with him that I had any kind of control. Part of the difficulty was in having already started to mourn. This was, for instance, the precise time in September when we had planned to return together to the place near Mallaig that I remembered with such nostalgia from childhood holidays. Aron would never see the view across to Skye now. He would never trail his hand in the water from the rowing boat with the outboard engine, or walk for miles through knee-high heather. There would be no more holidays—anywhere, just pain and the dying that progressed a little every minute.

There would be no more walks. No more of those discussions about films that went on far into the night. No more lovemaking, or did I dare to think of that? I can't remember. But worse than anything somehow, there would be no more ordinary living. No more fooling about with each other as we tried to get out of the flat on time in the mornings. No more arguments about our particular inability to share an umbrella without directing the rain down both our necks. Instead this barrack hospital, where life was geared to injections and temperature charts and checking the contents of bedpans and urine bottles. And after that, just nothing.

It was, I suppose, a hospital like many others. It had practically no civilised amenities at all. The only places that I frequented outside Aron's room were the single staff lavatory (which I was privileged to have the use of) and the room known as the sluice. Here there was generally at least one polythene bag containing urine and/or blood lying beside the sink, and I got as accustomed as the nurses to the sight of male patients walking about the ward with these bags attached to their persons.

Aron's room was a suntrap, and as the cruel summer persisted—there would be gold light now on the mountain tops, and clear blue-greens quite deep down in the sea—he lay there sweating helplessly and wishing away the last heat of the sun that he would ever know. But if I opened the window, battalions of wasps always swarmed in. There must have been a plague of them that year. I waged a savage war on them with an insecticide spray, and watched them slowly dying with a callousness that surprised me, for not long before I would have balked at killing even a fly.

From that first day I spent every minute I could with Aron. I went to the hospital as soon as I got up in the morning, and left only when the lights were going out in the ward. The worst thing was leaving him at night. There was just a thin partition between his room and the ward, and anyway I had to leave his door open so that the night nurses could hear him. I knew that for hours he lay awake listening to the coughs and groans and vomiting of all the sick old men outside. I knew too that he would have to feel very ill and desperate indeed before he asked for help or attention. He was an absolutely undemanding person. He automatically respected everybody else's right not to be bothered by his problems.

But most of all I hated leaving him simply because we had so little time left together. I wanted to be with him now for every minute that there was. I was madly in love. This was all that I had in the world, this last short time of Aron's company, and of course I grudged missing even a second of it. If friends offered to drive me to the hospital, I wanted them to do it at once. I thought it no kindness to offer me coffee or conversation or anything that would delay my departure. The rest of the world would always be there. Only Aron wouldn't.

Aron scarcely commented on his situation now, but he was the sort of person for whom hell is an institution, any institution. Military service had been the worst time in his life till now. Sometimes, in contemplating the awfulness of everything that surrounded his last days on earth, I thought it easily possible that I might lose my reason. After all, I shared most of my outlook on life with him. We were one spirit, as well as one flesh. What was happening to him was happening to me. How could I let it happen and not go mad?

My father used to come and meet me at the hospital when I was ready to go home. At first he met me for lunch as well, but after a few days I refused to leave Aron at lunchtime, and they gave me hospital meals in his room. I remember saying to my father that I thought I might go mad, and I don't think he really contradicted the idea. He mostly just listened to me, let me talk as wildly as I liked. I don't know what he did by himself all day. He must have exhausted the possibilities of browsing in bookshops. I regarded him as reasonably young and able to fend for himself, but he was actually over seventy then.

Sometime not long after the operation Aron's parents came to see him. When I took them into his room, he was obviously in considerable pain, but I didn't immediately hold his hand. We all tried to have an ordinary conversation, and Aron's mother alarmed me very much by mentioning my father in a way that could have aroused Aron's suspicions. Then I held his hand for a little, and everybody seemed to think this the best thing to do. Later I went away and left them on their own.

I remember, when they went back to Wales, seeing them on to a bus for the station. (I would have thought a taxi essential in such circumstances.) I told them not to think that they would never see Aron again, because they would. We were fighting and there would be a long time yet. I told them that I wanted to bring Aron home again before the end.

They nodded, apparently believing me.

'While there is life, there is hope,' said Aron's mother.

An odd thing was that Aron never asked anybody any questions. In the old days he had had a habit of saying 'Why are you looking like that?' He used to say it to me almost automatically if I just looked pensive, or if my expression noticeably altered in any way. Suddenly this had stopped. At first, in the little room, I was always waiting for it. When I thought my grief must be obvious, I would bury my face in the bedclothes as often as I dared. But the question never came, then or later. He never again repeated it.

I think the doctors and nurses were actually a little puzzled by his apparent lack of interest in the illness itself.

'Does he ask you any questions?' Dr. Lewis said to me a week or so after the operation.

'No.'

'He doesn't ask any of us either. He hasn't asked us anything,' he said in slightly surprised tones.

Maybe Aron asked no questions because he guessed the truth and wanted it to remain unspoken. Certainly I wanted it to remain unspoken now, and Aron could have sensed that too. But whatever the explanation for his reticence, my silence on this subject very soon ceased to seem like a lie. The diagnosis had quickly become something not needing to be talked about. It was the lesser of two truths. A favourite line of ours was from Jean Cocteau's valedictory film *Le Testament d'Orphée*: 'Faites semblant de pleurer, mes amis, puisque les poètes ne font que semblant d'être morts.' Pretend to weep, because poets only pretend to die. In the same way everything that might divide us, including death, seemed less real then than our love.

Aron's body, being a material thing, would conform to the scientists' prognosis, but Aron would only pretend to die.

* * *

The fact is that I arrived at the hospital feeling daily more happy at the prospect of being with him again. I looked forward to each reunion with as much plain excitement as I felt when we first knew each other ten years before.

One day when I arrived in the ward, the sister stopped me and said that I would have to go away until the afternoon. Mr. Warfield-Scrogge was doing a big teaching round with a group of post-graduate students and it wouldn't be convenient to have me around.

I think she had no idea that this would matter to me very much, because her manner had been almost off-hand. She had gone away before I had time to ask her precisely when I could come back. Practically in tears, I found one of the staff nurses and asked her how long the ward was closed to me. Then I slunk off home, where sorrow gradually turned to rage.

They thought they owned Aron, whom they couldn't help and couldn't cure. My presence there was just something that they condoned. It was a favour, not a right. All this was wrong. Aron belonged to me, not them. He needed me far more. It was I who gave him dignity and importance. It was for me that he was trying to stay alive. And he *was* trying to stay alive. There could be no doubt about it. He was fighting now, every inch of the way. I think it was probably then that I decided definitely that I had to get Aron out of the hospital, away from hospitals altogether. I had to bring him home. I must fight too.

Aron was in fact the only patient not included in Mr. Warfield-Scrogge's round that day. Instead a first-year student nurse gave him a blanket bath as part of her practical assessment. He could never have enough blanket baths because he was always hot and sweating and longing to be clean. So the morning actually went quite well for him.

I had given him a blanket bath myself once. I would have done it more often, in order to make myself useful, had it not been for the commotion it caused. Although there was running water in his room and the bed couldn't possibly have been seen by anyone in the ward, basins and screens had to be brought from the far corners of the place so that the procedure was conducted in the proper manner. Moreover, a time had to be selected when the assistant matron was unlikely to come round, because the assistant matron, according to everyone, was something of a prude. It certainly seemed that, far from helping by trying to do the thing ourselves, we were giving everybody more trouble, and Aron wouldn't have this. He went off the idea altogether after that.

The sister belonged to the Florence Nightingale tradition of nursing as it persists unaltered by changed times. She ruled her underlings with a rod of iron, treating them like schoolgirls or domestic servants, and yet taking for granted a professional dedication that would be highly prized in any other calling. She wouldn't hesitate, for instance, to reprimand a nurse, in front of the patients, for having her shoelace untied. She liked to see everybody always looking busy, clearing out cupboards or washing down the sluice, rather than simply standing talking to patients, which she regarded as a waste of time.

When Aron was out in the ward, the nurses stopped to chat to him only when the sister was off duty. Conversations with lonely or anxious patients weren't regarded as in any way part of a nurse's job. On the other hand, the arrangement of flowers was. The sister ordered the nurses to spend quite considerable periods of time on this, and got very angry if any withered blooms were allowed to remain in vases. Perhaps it was the flowers that I was always bringing for Aron that endeared me to her. Certainly, as time went on, she and I formed a reasonably good relationship in spite of having very little in common.

She had strongly religious leanings, and every Sunday morning she gave a troupe of evangelists the freedom of the ward. They sang hymns and said prayers before a captive audience of sick and suffering, among whom only the most rabid agnostic would have been foolish enough to give offence to the extent of asking to be wheeled away. Only the thoroughly mobile or those who, like Aron, had separate rooms, could without impropriety find themselves elsewhere at the time. The nurses all had to stop whatever they were doing, even if it were dressing a wound, and take part in the general thanksgiving.

I arrived one Sunday morning to find the service already in progress in the ward. To reach Aron, I would have had to cut right through it. I tiptoed into the nearest office, which happened to be the one belonging to the doctors. Dr. Lewis was standing there, staring dreamily at his desk, plainly doing nothing in particular.

'I'd hoped to get through before this began,' I whispered in explanation.

'Don't we all!' he responded.

'Haven't you found the back door?' he added. 'You go round the building and through the car park. You'd find it useful. It's at the same end of the ward as Aron's room.'

Every Tuesday morning Mr. Warfield-Scrogge, followed by a host of minions, did his regular ward round. You detected the difference almost as soon as you arrived on Tuesdays, the reverential hush. At the end of the round, coffee was served in the sister's office to the most important people, and fine bone china, quite unlike anything the patients ever drank from, came out for the occasion. I was sometimes, though not always, sent away to sit behind the flowers at the far end of the ward until the round was over. I rejoined Aron about the time that the nice coffee cups appeared.

I disliked being sent away because, apart from the obvious reasons, I imagined myself to be performing some kind of protective function by staying with Aron at such times. In fact, of course, the surgeon was every bit as protective about Aron as I was. He never took anyone other than the registrar or house surgeon into Aron's room with him. He was careful not to involve Aron in teaching sessions.

On one such round, when I was sitting at the other end of the ward, Mr. Warfield-Scrogge told Aron that he had received a letter from a director of Aron's firm, asking for particulars about his illness.

'Have I your permission to tell him about it?' he said to Aron.

Aron readily agreed. He was pleased to hear of the interest being taken in him.

I saw the whole thing in rather a different light. I felt that Mr. Warfield-Scrogge had no right to ask Aron a question, the meaning of which he was in no position to understand. I very much disliked the idea of Aron's employers knowing exactly what was wrong with him. I disliked it for all sorts of reasons but most of all, I think, for an intangible one. I felt that the surgeon's prognosis gained in certainty the more it was accepted and noised around. I knew what he had meant when he told me that it was wrong to predict exactly how long a patient had to live. By the same reasoning, it was really wrong to predict death positively at all. To do it was to kill Aron in our minds. To tell strangers about it was to kill him in the outside world. I determined to have it out with the surgeon before he left the ward.

I found him in the centre of an involved discussion near the door. The sister, who was standing on the outer fringe of this, asked me what I wanted and I told her.

'I think it's not fair,' I said. 'I should have been consulted. I'm the only one who understands what the question really means, and I don't want my husband's firm to know about him. The more people who know, the more difficult it's going to be. I'll always be afraid that somebody will make a slip.'

Actually I felt that I had reached a rather satisfactory position with Aron's firm. They understood that he was very ill, but only in the way that Aron understood it. I sent them medical certificates with notes that I wrote at his bedside. I remember being so proud of signing my married name on these. I don't think I had this feeling about my married name till then. Aron's courage had given me a new kind of pride in being his wife.

'I write to his firm regularly, and he sees all the letters,' I said. 'How will I manage if they know?'

'Shshsh . . .' said the sister, who was becoming increasingly agitated at the possibility of my outburst reaching the ears of the great man standing only a few yards away.

'Is it fair *not* to tell your husband's firm?' she said. 'They will need to make arrangements about the job, won't they?'

At this I became incensed.

'They know he won't be back for a long time. I write to them regularly, and I've made that quite clear. How can we be so sure he'll never work again. It's his job, and he's still alive. What if he were to hear that somebody else had got his job?'

'All right,' she said soothingly. 'All right, I'll tell Mr. Warfield-Scrogge how you feel. I'll tell him that you don't want Mr. Evans' firm to know. You'll find that there will be nothing to worry about.'

I decided to content myself with this. I don't know what happened afterwards. But the sister was right. There never was anything to worry about. As far as we were concerned, it was as if the question had never arisen.

5

Outwardly I was beginning to develop a certain composure now, except in relation to Mr. Warfield-Scrogge, whose easy assumption of authority I more and more resented. His intention to communicate with Aron's firm without consulting me was typical of the attitude I deplored. Obviously he discounted me altogether. But apart from that, no priest would surely have felt free to reveal such confidential information to others without the conscious permission of the person concerned. Any justification that there was seemed to me utterly materialistic. Aron was being regarded not as a person but as a unit, employable or otherwise, in the commercial world. If I had been paying for private treatment, would I have been consulted first about this? I don't know. I think there is a certain medical attitude that always assumes the right to decide everything for other people.

The hospital was Warfield-Scrogge territory as far as I was concerned. I was inhibited by it, and never very good at fighting there. I felt increasingly that getting Aron out of it might give us both a new lease of life. But I said very little about this to anyone.

I vaguely remember telling some of my friends in hurried phone calls. But I noticed, even then, that the possibility of getting Aron home for what brief time was left, made very little impression on them. Some of them were actually discouraging.

'You'd never manage. Isn't he better where he is?'

These were in general the people who reacted as if the end had come the moment they heard about it. It seemed not to occur to them at all how much the time between must matter to me. And yet it was right that it should matter. It's one thing to love someone when there aren't any problems and facts like death are so remote that almost no account is taken of them. But the real test of a relationship is what happens when substantial strain is put on it. Aron wasn't dead, and I had the chance, precariously held, to make him feel how profoundly he was loved before he went. The only peace that either of us could achieve seemed to me to depend on how much I was capable of giving to him then.

From the outset too he made it obvious how much he needed me. I remember thinking how terrible it would be if I got run over rushing to the hospital. He would have such a frightening death without me. I was always in a hurry outside the hospital, frantic to get there and frantic to return home in order to sleep enough to have some energy for him the next morning. I got wildly impatient waiting for buses or taxis. I used to walk out of shops if I wasn't served immediately. I had never felt so needed.

And all the time Aron was steadily recovering from the operation. The wound was healing very well, and by his own choice he was having less and less morphia injected into him. The nurse from Trinidad had made it clear to him that it was always better not to have an injection than to have one. He began trying to eat again, instead of existing only on fluids.

Then one day as I passed the sister's office, she called me in.

'What do you think about taking him home?' she said.

'Could I?' I asked. The offer was so sudden, so incredible that it almost took my breath away. I had no idea that anyone in the hospital was seriously thinking along these lines.

'Yes, I think so. Once we get him on his feet a little.'

For a moment I was speechless. This was marvellous if she

really meant it, if she really knew that it could work. Then I said:

'What about the injections?'

'Oh, that's quite easy. You can give him those in tablet form.'

Dr. Lewis was sitting beside her, and I looked at him for confirmation. He was swinging backwards on his chair, balancing himself with one toe, his hands in his pockets. He just smiled and nodded. I began to smile then too.

'I'd love to take him home,' I said, still conveying only a fraction of my real feelings on the subject. Actually I wanted this so much that I had to be sure they weren't being over-optimistic before I started banking on it absolutely. 'But could I manage all right?' I added.

'Why not?' said the sister. 'You have another bed that you could sleep on?'

'Yes. Yes, certainly. I could move the studio couch into the same room.'

'And is the bathroom on the same floor?'

'Yes, it is. It's on the same floor.'

'Well I don't think there would be any difficulties really. I'm sure he would be much happier at home.'

That was about all that was said then, but it was enough to give me unbelievable hope. I thought, however, that I would have to consult Mr. Warfield-Scrogge about it first. So I made an appointment to see him. I came to the point at once.

Mr. Warfield-Scrogge regarded me rather grimly.

'What happened when your husband first attempted to eat yesterday?' he said

I had to admit that Aron had been sick.

'That will happen more and more,' he said. 'You must realise how ill he is. He will never be able to eat properly again.'

This pronouncement nearly made me cry. Mr. Warfield-Scrogge could undermine me so easily. Immediately I began to feel defeated by the ghastly physical details of the disease he could claim to know so much more about than I. I stopped thinking straight, as I always do when confronted by people like this—people absolutely confident they can assess others in a matter of minutes. I knew the way he assessed me. He thought I had very little character or personality.

Reinforced by my stricken silence, he pressed his point.

'Has he shown any inclination to get out of bed?' he said.

He hadn't. I wondered for the first time why this was.

'He'll never be any better than he is now,' the surgeon declared. 'Surely it will be easier for you both if he stays here.'

I felt somehow that Mr. Warfield-Scrogge had implied immediately after the operation that Aron would never be any better than he was then. If so, he had been wrong. But I couldn't be sure of anything really. I knew I ought to argue, prove the strength of my feelings. But how? On what basis? I was defeated by something that he obviously meant as sympathy. He possibly still believed that I didn't really want this much responsibility.

I knew now that if Aron stayed in hospital, I would feel for the rest of my life that I had failed him. Yet there seemed no way of saying this to a man like Mr. Warfield-Scrogge. I could only have said it to someone sufficiently sensitive to appreciate at once that I wasn't being hysterical. Any display of strong emotion would, I felt, be regarded by him as hysteria. It would suggest to him that I wasn't really capable of handling the situation I so much wanted to bring about. And so I couldn't possibly say how much seemed to me to depend on bringing Aron home.

Another obstacle to communication was that Mr. Warfield-Scrogge was obviously unaware of the realities of hospital life as they struck us, the drabness and the ugliness of it all. He saw only the best china, and everybody standing to attention when he came into the ward. He had no idea what it was really like there for Aron and for me. But this was something it would have seemed ungrateful and insulting to point out.

I left him in such a state of desperation that I was terrified of its effect on Aron. It was really as if I had been told the prognosis for the first time all over again. I paced up and down the ward, afraid of facing Aron in tears and afraid of not facing him for very much longer.

Seeking refuge in the sluice, I asked a staff nurse for an aspirin. She advised me against this—God knows why. Perhaps, the system being what it was, she couldn't easily have given it to me on her own authority. Anyway, it hardly mattered. I was simply marking time until I felt up to going back to Aron. When I finally went back, he made no comment whatsoever on my still obvious agitation.

The Indian summer ironically continued. Every day was bathed in a kind of awful beauty. The gardens remained lush and green, and people who stayed at home all day were virtually living in them. Children's toys and bicycles were still lying outside in the late evening, and doors and windows were left constantly open in a way that reminded me of the continent. The rose bushes that we had planted only about a spring ago, went on and on producing blooms. There were always roses to pick for Aron. I used to notice every detail of their petals and their leaves. There would be more of them again next summer and the summer after. Nature would go on repeating itself whether I paid any attention to it or not. But Aron wouldn't be there however much I tried to hold him with my love. Aron wouldn't see next season's crop of roses. It was like one of those adolescent dreams I used to have about harrowing, romantic situations. But it wasn't a dream, this desperate need to surround him with as much love and beauty as his world could hold, to give him something worth having before it was all over. The Indian summer that I found so painful because it had come too late for Aron, at least gave him roses. It had that much generosity.

I used to try to look good too. I went to the hairdresser regularly for the first time in my life, although I grudged every minute of the time it took. I sometimes wondered how the assistants would have reacted if they'd known. What if I'd asked them to hurry because my husband was dying and there was very little time left? Might they have thought up a particularly flattering style instead of simply seeing that I conformed to current fashion? But no, it was impossible. People don't say things like that, at least I don't. It would have been too dramatic, the first time maybe that such a thing had happened. None of this, I thought, had ever happened before. I was living in a world that didn't and couldn't exist for other people.

Long before our roses ended, crysanthemums began to appear in the shops. I took those to him too. I remember going back once with a huge bunch of them, all flame and gold. While I was arranging them, I accidentally knocked the head off one. Without thinking, I put the crysanthemum head on the sheet just under Aron's chin. Then, instantly aghast at the image I had created, I snatched it away again. Aron didn't notice anything; he merely suggested finding a small receptacle for the severed flower. Beautiful things just pleased him. There was no likelihood of them hurting at the same time as they so often did with me.

Ten days after the operation the stitches had been removed. The wound was in good condition. Now orders came from the sister to the nursing staff to get Aron on his feet again. This was a brutal business, necessarily. A male nurse came to supervise Aron's first steps. After a moment or two in the upright position, Aron fainted. Then he vomited. Then he went back to bed.

It was a start, however alarming. After that he got up and walked a little more each day. There was no more vomiting the second time. Also he stopped having injections altogether, and went on to palfium tablets instead.

Although Dr. Lewis and the nursing staff saw Aron every day, Mr. Warfield-Scrogge saw him only once or twice a week. He nonetheless based his impression of Aron's progress on precisely what he found the days he came to the ward. On one such day, about three weeks after the operation, Aron was feeling rather sick. He had been keen to sit up, and walk around a bit, every other day of the preceding week. But that day he just lay on his back, looking yellow and ill.

Mr. Warfield-Scrogge summed up the situation at a quick glance. He decided that more sedation was needed, and prescribed morphia injections again. These were to be given in addition to more palfium tablets. I was there when he did it, and saw all this being written up on Aron's card. Aron was going to regard it as a very backward step, because he knew that the injections and the pills were for the pain and weren't otherwise beneficial.

I went to see the sister afterwards, and asked her what was to be done to prevent Aron from worrying. I was certain that he didn't need all this sedation, but if the sister didn't argue with Mr. Warfield-Scrogge, how could I?

'Tell him they are different injections,' she said.

'But he's to have more tablets too.'

'Tell him that both the tablets and the injections are new.'

I nodded and left the room. What else was there to do? The only person to tackle really was Mr. Warfield-Scrogge, and I wasn't capable of that. Everything he said seemed calculated to make me lose my nerve. Then an unfortunate thing happened. I met the surgeon accidentally in the ward.

'How do you find your husband today?' he asked gravely.

'Not very well,' I confessed.

He nodded.

'I'm afraid he's very ill indeed.' He paused, weighing his words. 'I think,' he said, 'that if there are any relatives who would like to see him, it would probably be advisable for you to contact them within a week.'

A week! Was it as bad as that? Could it possibly be as bad as that? Should I call his parents back already? I had told them that they would see Aron again, and they believed me. If Mr. Warfield-Scrogge was right, they would have to be told. They would have to come again soon. I must act for Aron, the way Aron would want.

Even as I was standing there in the hideous, bleak ward, I

could see us all playing fruit machines together in pouring rain on Mumbles pier. It was no time ago really, and yet whole worlds away. Christ, to be back among such ordinary things! I decided that Mr. Warfield-Scrogge was wrong. I told Aron's parents nothing of his latest alarm.

But the repercussions of the surgeon's visit didn't end there. Later in the day, an Irish male nurse, ignorant of the line to be adopted, presented one of the tablets to Aron, describing it as his usual one.

Aron pointed out that if it was his usual one, he wasn't supposed to be having it any more. The nurse immediately lost his temper, and started to shout out that he was merely acting on instructions. He said he was sick of being criticised and disbelieved. Aron could take the pill, or not, as he wished. The nurse must have had a bad day already, because he got more and more worked up, bellowing and storming about the injustice of everything. All through it Aron just lay there looking puzzled. I could hardly stand it.

'Please,' I said. 'Please remember he's ill.' At which the nurse stamped angrily out of the room.

* * *

The next morning when Dr. Lewis came to see him, Aron complained that he could hardly raise his head from the pillow.

'I'm so drugged,' he said.

'What's he on?' the doctor asked the staff nurse. Taking the treatment card from her, he crossed off the injections and added suppositories to be given as an anti-emetic.

'If you feel sick, just ask for the suppositories,' he told Aron.

Certainly if Dr. Lewis hadn't taken Aron off morphia when he did, any chance of his ever leaving hospital would have been lost for ever. The young doctor was on our side. He was standing up for life, whatever the odds. Aron had already benefited from his friendship. Often at night, when I had gone, Dr. Lewis would talk to him for hours. He had the courage to be involved. And it is an emotional risk to be involved with the dying. The nursing system is hedged in with safeguards to protect nurses from taking it unnecessarily. It's really quite difficult for a nurse to become deeply involved with any one patient. Quite apart from the fact that she is likely to be moved frequently from one ward to another, she has so many practical things to do. It's inadvisable for her to allow a patient to become dependent on her because any day or any minute she may have to be elsewhere.

As Aron became more mobile we both saw more of the other patients in the ward. There was a youngish man with ulcers who used to regale us with all the details of his illness and his treatment. He also envied Aron his privileges, and was tactless enough to comment on them.

'How do you get a room on your own, and your wife allowed to stay here all day?' he said.

But even this appeared not to worry Aron. He just smiled and shrugged. Of course, one could easily attribute our special treatment to the unacknowledged class distinctions still prevalent everywhere in Britain today. Ineffectual as I was in my relationship with Mr. Warfield-Scrogge, we must nonetheless have qualified as members of the educated minority who get more cushioning than the rest. We were privileged. Nobody else in that ward had a room to himself, although there was another, older patient that I knew of, who was an equally hopeless case. His wife visited him in the surroundings that I regarded as intolerable for Aron and myself. I used to think this dreadful. Conceivably so did they.

One or two of the other patients guessed about Aron. There was an elderly man, some sort of academic I should think (he discussed Greek and Latin literature with Aron) who plainly knew. He made it clear to me that he was desperately sorry.

'I'm old,' he said. 'I've had my life. Sometimes I think they waste their time going on patching me up. I wish they could do something for him instead.'

It occurs to me now that he talked like this to Aron too,

because Aron repeated some of it to me. I wonder if Aron really knew, even then. Whether he did or not, he was tremendously determined not to give in. It was inspiring, the effort that he made to walk as far as the back door and then to negotiate the two or three stone steps down to the car park outside. Being in the open air again was something of a triumph. It tired him out completely, so that afterwards he just lay on his bed for a long time looking contented. The sort of rest he had now was more natural, much less dependent on drugs.

Each day he walked a little farther, and his activities didn't pass unnoticed. Once when we were walking outside, I saw Mr. Warfield-Scrogge watching from the window of the sister's room. Later that day the surgeon paid us a surprise visit.

'If you like,' he said to Aron, 'if you feel well enough, you can go home for a day or a weekend sometime now.'

The effect of this statement was miraculous. There was no stopping Aron after that. He walked as far as he could go inside the hospital grounds. He said almost nothing about it, but it was obvious that all his energy was concentrated on not losing the opportunity of getting out for even a day. Or perhaps, like me, he knew that it wasn't going to be only a day. With any luck at all it was going to be much longer even than a weekend. Certainly from the first I saw it as my chance to get him out of hospital altogether, my only chance.

Leaving him at night was getting worse, rather than better, now that he was off regular injections. Before I left, he used to get two palfium tablets as night sedation. At other times, he was written up for one palfium tablet four hourly, as necessary. But these appeared not to be laid on automatically during the night. If he wanted one at night there was always an extremely long delay (over an hour on one occasion) before he got it. This was because the night staff had to refer to a night sister for the keys of the cupboard containing drugs listed under the dangerous drugs act. The night sister had several wards to cover, and could sometimes be in another wing of the hospital at the time. The nurses on the ward were still training, and had no authority to give a drug like this even when it was prescribed for a patient. They were very sorry. They used to offer Aron soluble codeine, and cups of tea, and sit beside him if they possibly could. The only thing they couldn't give him was the specialised treatment that he was ostensibly in hospital to get.

Sometimes the soluble codeine worked, but Aron hardly ever got through a night without needing at least one palfium tablet and I thought the situation pretty intolerable. I discussed it with the sister, who agreed that it would be a good idea to leave a tablet for Aron on his locker last thing at night. She said she would see that this was done in future. But it couldn't be done. As she must have known quite well, there is a rule forbidding it. Drugs of this kind cannot be left lying around. The night staff adhered to the rule, and things continued in the same way night after night.

I began to feel the strain of it badly. My own sleeping pill wasn't enough to prevent me from lying awake at night wondering if Aron was getting his tablet when he needed it. If he came home, I would have control of these tablets. It would put an end to this.

It was now more or less understood between us that, all continuing well, Aron would come home the following weekend, the first weekend he could in fact. That would be about four weeks after the operation. Aron himself had asked the sister, and she had agreed to this. The registrar had also looked in and given his permission. Even at this stage I said very little about it to anybody. Too much was at stake.

On Thursday evening, at the time I usually left, Aron was still waiting for his night sedation. I liked to see him get this before I went away, so eventually I went and asked about it. After a while, a nurse brought him one tablet instead of the usual two. Apparently only the one tablet had been left out for him, and now the keys were away with the night sister who was on her rounds. A delay was inevitable.

I waited. It was getting very late, and I had intended to

67

start on preparations for Aron's home-coming when I got back that night. To me it was incomprehensible that things should be organised so badly in the hospital. How could the rules be so ridiculous as to allow this kind of situation to arise at all, let alone recur night after night? In the end, out of kindness, one of the nurses succeeded in persuading me to go.

'He'll get his tablet,' she said. 'I'll see that he gets it. Don't worry.'

Certainly I was far too worked up to be doing Aron any good by staying there, so I said goodnight. Before I left, however, I whispered that, if I could help it, this wouldn't happen again.

'Tomorrow,' I said, 'tomorrow instead of Saturday, if they let me, I'm taking you home. There's only tonight until you come home. Only tonight.'

6

Clive Arundel, the friend who first introduced us to each other, was waiting in the hospital hallway to take me home that night. He had made his name in Fleet Street in recent years. He now wrote a syndicated column on show business, and interviewed film people on television. He was about six feet tall with shaggy eyebrows and thick black hair already greying at the temples, which made him more attractive than he used to be. Also, no doubt as a direct result of being so popular and so much in demand, he was gayer and more amusing than before.

But we saw far less of him. He rationed his time rather carefully now. And we felt, perhaps wrongly, that we interested him less too. It seemed to us that on his recent visits it wasn't us he came for. It was our news, our possessions, our latest books and records, any links that we had with the swinging, meaningless world of 'with it' people and 'with it' things. As soon as we had covered all that, he had a maddening habit of springing to his feet with a familiar cry of 'Well, I must go.'

This certainly wasn't because he felt important. In fact, I think he usually deferred to Aron, came to him for qualities that he appreciated as rare. Perhaps it was a kind of anxiety that made him always in such a rush. Success, especially in his line, is such a chancy business that maybe you really have to organise your life down to the last detail to keep up with it. Also Clive seemed really none too happy. For one thing he was never going to marry and yet, I think, wanted to be the sort of person who might. This way, there was no time left to stop and think and maybe brood.

Anyway, it must have thrown his timetable considerably that I was so late that night. In fact, I dashed out once to tell him I was coming in case he gave up hope and went away. But he was very charming, and said nothing whatsoever about time. What he did say was that his smooth sports car had broken down, and that he had brought his motor bike instead. Physical comforts matter quite a lot when you are already feeling somewhat shaken. The soles of my shoes were far too thin for riding on the machine, and the powerful engine seemed to throb right through my body. I arrived home literally reeling with tiredness.

My father looked enormously glad to see us, and immediately offered us whisky, which helped. It was pleasant for him to have somebody like Clive to talk to, because so much of the time there was nobody, and I provided rather cheerless company in the short times when I was there. For a moment we all sat down. But I had determined it would be for only a moment. I set an even higher value on my time than Clive did at that juncture. There wouldn't be anyone as strong as Clive around before tomorrow, and I needed furniture moved. As I swallowed the whisky, I was deciding exactly what the priorities were.

'A terrible business this!' my father said.

'Terrible!' said Clive. 'And it's going to be worse before it's better too.'

Somehow this last remark enraged me. I had just told Clive that Aron was coming home. I thought the news made very little impression on him, but it really sounded as if it hadn't penetrated at all.

'Oh no, it won't,' I said, then turning to my father, 'Aron's coming home tomorrow.' It was such a wonderful thing to be able to say, but nobody gave the slightest sign of jubilation.

'No, no.' My father spoke wearily, like one who had been

alone all day with just this single thought of Aron dying, and nothing that anybody could do about it. He was very fond of Aron.

'How do you mean "no, no"?' I snapped. 'The whole thing's decided. I'm bringing him home tomorrow.'

My father looked bewildered.

'Mr. Warfield-Scrogge won't let you,' he said. 'He won't allow it.'

'How do you mean? He has allowed it. He said that Aron could come home for a weekend, and his registrar confirmed that this weekend would be all right.'

I would have been so happy if someone, just for a moment, had rejoiced with me. But instead the two men sat there with long, sad faces—disbelieving, almost disapproving of my miracle.

'I'm going to measure the wardrobe,' I said abruptly. 'Can you spare a minute to help me move it when you've finished your drink, Clive?'

'Yes of course,' he said quickly.

I went away and surveyed our bedroom—the bedroom that belonged to Aron and me. I wanted to make it look as much like a bed-sitting room as possible. This meant moving the wardrobe into the spare bedroom, if there was room for it there, and bringing in the studio couch instead. The flat was on two floors, and the studio couch was downstairs at the moment. There would have to be room for the wardrobe in the spare room really, because with that mirror down the front of it, it couldn't possibly stay where it was. Aron would see himself every time he sat up in bed. He would see what was happening to him.

I emptied the entire contents of the wardrobe on to the bed. There were some papers lying in the bottom of it. Lifting them out to put them in a more suitable place, I noticed a little card on the top. It was from the mass X-ray service and it said, 'I am pleased to tell you that in my opinion your recent X-ray examination was satisfactory.' It was addressed to Aron. He always had regular chest X-rays. (I had never had one in my life. I think I was actually too scared that something might be discovered if I did.) It was dated less than a year before.

The awful thing was that the primary carcinoma in Aron's case had apparently been in the lung. When Dr. Lewis told me this, I exclaimed about the X-rays. But apparently it was quite in order that nothing should have been detected that way. The cancer would have had to go much farther in the lung before it showed.

'REMEMBER—' it said at the bottom of the card in capital letters 'THE EARLIER FOUND, THE MORE EASILY CURED.' Aron was continually going to the doctor, especially about his catarrh. There was nothing else he could have done in the normal course of events in order to have had the disease detected sooner. I threw the thing into a cupboard, and called Clive.

He appeared immediately, and asked what he was to do. I explained about the wardrobe. It was going to be difficult to get it round the tiny landing without falling downstairs or getting stuck. We heaved and pushed until it appeared to be fairly firmly jammed across the landing.

'It won't go any farther,' Clive said at once.

It amazed me how easily he gave in. I insisted that it would, and in fact it did. With a little more effort we moved it into the other room. We also carried the studio coach upstairs before Clive left.

Much later I learned why Clive showed a certain lack of enthusiasm about moving the furniture. Apparently, when I was upstairs, my father told him that, whatever I said, Aron would definitely not be coming home.

Without my knowledge, my father had gone to see Mr. Warfield-Scrogge, who had assured him that Aron would remain in hospital. I don't know exactly when this was, but it mystified me afterwards as much as the ensuing events must have mystified my father at the time. The only explanation is that we had won a greater victory than we realised, Aron and I.

Presumably Mr. Warfield-Scrogge never actually believed us capable of effectively carrying through our dream of escape.

*　　*　　*

The day of Aron's homecoming was as beautiful and mellow as all the days that had gone before. The mid-October sun made the autumnal colours glow. Aron had always loved the autumn, its mixture of sadness and fulfilment, ripeness and decay. He liked to walk in autumn woods and feel nostalgic. He loved the world for what it was, accepted and enjoyed a much wider range of sensations than I did. I used to regret the autumn. I wanted the perpetual promise of spring, at least I did until I walked through autumn woods with Aron.

I arrived at the hospital earlier than usual that morning. The floors were being cleaned and Aron's bed, together with all the furniture from his room, was out in the corridor of the main ward. There amid the roar of vacuum cleaners he lay, flat on his back, reading a thriller. From a long way off I could tell by the angle of his arm that he was all right. He was all right, and he would be coming home. The moment that this was positively established, I went into a whirl of activity. All the preparations that I hadn't dared to make in case they should prove unnecessary, were crammed into a few hours.

'He's coming home today.' That was all I could think:

> 'Quick now, here, now always—
> Ridiculous the waste sad time
> Stretching before and after.'

'He's coming home today,' I shouted to Jennie as I rushed into the flat with a pile of shopping. I think she must have gone straight out to a florist, because later an enormous bunch of dahlias arrived to welcome Aron: huge, blazing flowers that lit up the whole room.

He wanted to go home in Irma and Dylan's old Rover, and Irma had offered to take him in it. But I was uncertain at first about the wisdom of it, and asked the sister if an ambulance might not be better.

'Knowing the way these ambulance drivers go,' she said dryly. 'I think he'd be more comfortable in your friends' car.'

I phoned Irma, who arranged to come for us in the afternoon. Then back at the hospital I had a final chat with the sister.

'If everything goes all right,' she said, 'you know that there's no need for him to come back on Monday. He can stay at home.'

'Yes,' I said, because I did know this. 'How long can he stay?'

'As long as you're managing to cope.'

'How long will I be able to cope?'

'There may be nothing very difficult. It could go on like this for quite a long time.' She paused for a moment, and then she said, 'We had a boy here once—he was younger than your husband, but in much the same condition. He went on like this for two years.'

'Two years!' I exclaimed, new vistas suddenly opening up in front of me.

'He went home and his parents looked after him. He took codeine most of the time. Of course, we can't expect anything like this length of time for Mr. Evans, but he may have quite a while yet, especially if he takes as little palfium as possible. You might perhaps try codeine some of the time.

'It will make such a difference for him to be at home,' she went on. 'He is the sort of patient who ought to be at home. This is something that only you can do for him, you know. You will be so glad later on. Years afterwards you will be glad when you remember it.'

I looked away. Of course, I knew all this. I was just so scared of failing that I had never dared to make it clear to anybody how much I knew it.

'What will happen at the end?' I half whispered.

'Nothing will happen,' she said. 'In the last days he will

probably sink into a coma, but by then I expect we will have him back here.'

I hoped very much that this wouldn't be the case, but I said nothing.

'The thing to remember is that when people are ill they don't want to be bothered with questions and decisions,' she said. 'You must make all his decisions for him now. You must take charge.'

I went back to Aron who had himself made the decision to come out of hospital. For it was in fact he, not I, who asked the permission of the sister and registrar. It would probably be his last decision; it must be one that he would never regret.

'The sister told me I needn't come back on Monday,' he said.

'When did she say this?' I was surprised that she should have mentioned it to Aron before discussing it with me.

'While you were looking for her, I think.'

'She's just told me the same.'

'Am I going to be all right?' Aron said, suddenly apprehensive. I knew what he was thinking; it was in my mind too. He was leaving a kind of shelter, a kind of security, and he was very ill. I took the hand that he stretched out to me, and held it very tightly.

'Yes,' I said firmly. 'You'll be all right.'

He smiled, relaxed, turned on the transistor radio that my father and I had bought for him during one of those recent, rushed lunch hours that now seemed very long ago. Perhaps it was going to be all right, I thought. Perhaps it was just a matter of sounding thoroughly confident.

A little later Mr. Warfield-Scrogge looked in.

'Now,' he said firmly, glancing from one of us to the other but concentrating on Aron, 'promise me that if there's any trouble, any trouble at all, you will come straight back here.'

Aron nodded.

'And on Monday,' the surgeon added, 'on Monday at the latest I expect to see you back in this bed.' After a few more words he vanished.

'The sister and Mr. Warfield-Scrogge don't seem to feel the same way about it,' Aron remarked after he'd gone. 'He came in here while you were away, and talked for quite a long time.'

'Everyone seems to come here while I'm away,' I said. 'What did he say?'

'Oh, he said that going home would put more of a strain on you than I realised. He seemed concerned about you.'

Just then we noticed the sister and Mr. Warfield-Scrogge walking up and down the car park outside the window, deep in discussion. They seemed to be not entirely in agreement.

'Perhaps they're arguing about us,' said Aron, sounding rather pleased at the idea.

I have always felt sure they were arguing about us. I used to imagine how the conversation possibly went.

'I've told young Evans to be sure to be back on Monday,' says the surgeon in the peremptory tones that he reserves for the discussion of cases like this, cases that his impotence to cure makes him feel most deeply hurt and angry about.

'Oh! Well, I've told both of them that he needn't come back,' she says.

'My God! I think you've made a big mistake there. She can't cope with a situation like this. I'm not sure she even accepts it. I'm not sure she realises what's going to happen.'

'That's what she said herself after you upset her the other day. She seems to think you don't believe she's grasped the facts.'

'Upset her? How did I upset her? By telling her the truth?'

'She said you told her the end might come in about a week.'

'Well! If it alarms her so much to be told a thing like that, how can she manage what she's trying to do?' he protests. 'It would hit her very badly if she failed, you know. Very badly indeed.'

But perhaps the conversation went quite differently. Perhaps the surgeon described again what he had seen in the operating theatre. This had obviously been so appalling that it surprised him that Aron could live with it at all. The sister, on the other hand, was accustomed to watching patients clinging impossibly to life. She knew from long experience at the bedside how very powerful the will to live can be.

The thing I doubt if they discussed, the thing that nobody ever really discussed, was how exactly I *would* cope. From this point of view, you might think I would have been put in touch with the medical social worker some time before. But Mr. Warfield-Scrogge was the kind of surgeon who never called in the medical social worker unless his patients or their relatives specifically requested it. He knew that he could cope better with every situation himself. I think I was aware that medical social workers existed, but I was uncertain of their function and made no attempt to see one on my own behalf. So from the beginning there was really no link between the hospital and home.

The sister knew only that the flat was suitable, that Aron would be on the same floor as the bathroom. She had no idea whether or not I would have any help. Nobody had asked me whether I had relatives or friends who were prepared to do the shopping and liaise between us and the outside world. Nobody even seemed to have made contact with our doctor, let alone the district nurse or anybody else outside the hospital in a position to help us to maintain a kind of independence. And so perhaps it was a romantic notion to think that the sister and surgeon were arguing about us at all. They were probably debating some new, more urgent case. We were probably more or less forgotten already.

The fact is that we were going out on our own, and if for any reason, however minor, we failed to make a success of it, our only alternative course of action was to come back. I wished I had formed a happier impression of Dr. Sciberas. But it was inconceivable that she, or anybody else, could fail to be as co-operative as possible with things as they stood now.

*　　*　　*

Our last hour in the hospital: I adjusted the angle of a flower in a vase beside the window.

'We'll leave all the flowers here,' I said. 'Perhaps we should start packing. What will we need?'

'My radio anyway,' said Aron. 'You decide what else.'

'There isn't much,' I said, looking at the contents of his locker. 'I can really pack it in a minute.'

This is an odd thing about being in hospital, how little people seem to need there. All the material possessions with which they normally surround themselves, and which they once regarded as vital to their well-being, get whittled down to a toilet bag and a shaving kit. I put the few essentials into a zip bag.

A staff nurse came in and handed me the medicines for Aron to take home. There were more palfium tablets than I had ever believed possible I would see at a single glance. Just to look at the fat little transparent container of them filled me with joy. Ever since, that kind of pill bottle has carried with it special associations for me—associations of copiousness, liberation, relief from pain.

'There are quite a lot here,' said the staff nurse, 'but try to take as few as possible. The fewer you can manage with the better.'

This was the other side of it, the knowledge that these drugs meant death as well as life. I knew the tightrope balance that had to be preserved as long as possible between the two. I also knew I could maintain it better than anybody else. I cared more than anybody else, and I had studied Aron's reactions to these tablets minutely. I had noticed, for instance, that if he had to wait too long for one, as happened often in the hospital, he went beyond the point where it was any use in alleviating the pain. He then needed another very soon after, and the total dose over a day was likely to be increased without a corresponding reduction in pain.

I knew the pain. There was no danger of my encouraging Aron to take more analgesics than he needed. I knew when the pain was bad and when it was less bad, simply by being with him. I intended to use this knowledge in administering the drugs. It was a much better guide than a treatment card that said four hourly or two hourly as necessary.

As soon as the staff nurse left the room, Aron said he would like a tablet there and then.

'What!' I exclaimed. 'You should have asked her for it. They'll go mad if they see me giving you one of these here.'

Actually he hadn't had one for hours because the whole programme had broken down that day, but he was so buoyed up by the prospect of going home that he hadn't noticed this till now.

When Irma drove into the car park, there were no nurses around anywhere. The patient who used to envy Aron his privileges but seemed now not to notice them providing he could pour out all his troubles to him, became quite agitated about this, and finally dashed off in search of somebody. He came back with the male nurse who had supervised Aron's first steps when he got up. The nurse took the zip bag from me. I took the radio from Aron, and we all went out into the sunshine.

I kept looking back, expecting something to happen, I'm not sure what. An enormous ceremonial farewell, or a curt order to relinquish this wild dream of freedom and come back at once. But it seemed as if our exit was to be one of those triumphs that pass almost completely unobserved. In fact, the absence of medical and nursing staff made it seem even a little furtive, like escaping from prison while the warders have temporarily turned their backs.

Aron and I sat side by side in the back seat of the Rover. On our wedding day too, for some odd reason, there had been a need to fight back tears. We passed the familiar shopfront near the hospital, the Georgian house with its red ivy on the wall. But this time I scarcely noticed even my own landmarks. I was keeping up a casual conversation with Irma, so that Aron wouldn't have to talk. It took so much out of him to be sociable. Then at last in a kind of tumult of pain and happiness all mixed up together, we arrived at the flat.

'Welcome home!' my father said. We were all standing in the living room. 'Your mother is on her way here,' he told me. 'She's coming on the night train.'

'What luck!' said Aron. 'She couldn't have timed it better.' He seemed actually to think that the whole thing was coincidence, that my mother just happened to be coming the day he happened to arrive home. Waves of relief were washing over me. Aron at home, and now my mother coming at least to tide us over the crucial first day or two.

'Do you want me to stay and chat, or leave you to get on?' said Irma.

I looked at Aron, who was still wearing his pyjamas and dressing gown. The sister had advised me not to let him waste energy by changing into ordinary clothes. Besides, he might have been alarmed to discover, by trying on his clothes, exactly how much weight he had lost in hospital. He looked very tired indeed. The journey had used up practically all the strength he had. It was the last supreme effort, for which he had been screwing himself up for days. He probably couldn't have done it without something of the instinct that animals have, the instinct to come home to die.

'We'd better go straight upstairs,' I said. So after we'd all thanked her, Irma went away.

Aron wouldn't let us help him to climb the stairs. He did it by himself, very slowly, step by step. And when he reached our bed, he fell totally exhausted on to it.

'What comfort!' he said. 'What comfort!' and closed his eyes.

7

While Aron was in hospital I was always looking back, brooding over past happiness, wishing myself in another time as well as another place. Now all that changed. I started to live entirely in the present. There was something to fight for here and now, something the more precious in that it couldn't be taken for granted and couldn't last.

Of course there was far more physical comfort at home. The hospital was noisy day and night, the bed hard, the food coarse and unsuitable for invalids. (The biggest, greasiest beefburgers I ever saw were served, once or twice weekly, to the patients in that surgical ward.) Really everything about the place was ugly, and there wasn't any peace. But the difference was far more than this. Right from the start the whole quality of Aron's life seemed to be transformed.

In hospital, for instance, he read nothing but thrillers— Michael Innes, Raymond Chandler, Patricia Highsmith, Nicolas Freeling, Simenon, Nicholas Blake, Andrew Garve, Hammond Innes—an endless string of them. Several friends had been kept busy providing a constant supply of the best they could find. Aron had never gone in for thrillers much till then. But in hospital they seemed to act on him like a drug. They were a drug, I suppose, an easy escape route from reality.

When he came home he didn't need them anymore. He just stopped reading them at once, and took up his former interests: music, literature, philosophy, politics, cricket, jazz. He read history and prehistory, browsed through Virgil's *Eclogues*: 'Sing on then, since we are seated on soft grass, and the year is at its loveliest, with growing crops in every field, fruit coming on every tree, and all the woods in leaf.' He was himself again, stretching his mind the way he used to stretch it, enjoying at least some of the things he had always enjoyed.

And I had done this. I had done it by myself. I had snatched this little extra piece of actual life for him, when otherwise there would have been nothing. Just death and nothing: 'a bracelet of bright hair about the bone'.

The decay and dissolution of his firm, warm body was really only half the horror. The worst thing, the thing impossible to accept or even grasp, was the extermination of his mind, the idea that all those intricate and subtle connections between his thinking self and the animate world around him would be extinguished too. Ludicrous to believe that this abomination of waste made any sense! And so you fought it by making the impressions and connections richer still, by helping him to go on thinking, remembering, communicating, loving, until the very last:

> 'Break in the sun till the sun breaks down,
> And death shall have no dominion.'

Sometimes the situation, in all its aspects, was almost explicit. He was like a drowning man in the moment of recapturing the vision of his entire life. When he asked for Neville Cardus's autobiography, for instance, it was because it was a book he had always meant to read again. A lot of it is very like him, at least like him at the time he first went up to Oxford, I think.

'It is in the arts,' Cardus concludes, 'that I have found the only religion that is real and, once found, omnipresent . . . If I know that my Redeemer liveth it is not on the church's testimony, but because of what Handel affirms. As Jowett put it to Margot: "My dear child, you must believe in God in spite of what the clergy may tell you".'

I didn't read poetry then. I didn't read anything. The only details on which I could concentrate were those connected with looking after Aron. But all the lines already in my head acquired a relevance to living they never had before. They weren't a consolation. There was no consolation. But they were a kind of strength: 'for better for worse, for richer for poorer, in sickness and in health, to love and to cherish, till death us do part.' That's poetry—something so true in itself that its religious context is irrelevant. I remember pacing up and down the sickroom with echoes of it fighting the pain. Even at a time like this there are words that won't disintegrate, won't give in:

'Though lovers be lost love shall not;
And death shall have no dominion.'

From childhood I had been haunted by a fear of cancer, and also a fear of death. One of the things that makes cancer so terrifying is that it is life before it becomes death. It is life gone mad. The younger its victim, the more rapidly are life cells and death cells regenerated, the swifter the death. We have no knowledge of the process that governs the normal divisions of cells, and cancer is an abnormal division of cells. Consequently in order to find a cure for it (as opposed to simply killing or cutting out affected tissue) we have to discover more about the nature of life itself.

I think the only way to rid yourself of any fear is to confront it directly. Both death and cancer are very common fears, but in our society it is actually difficult to confront either directly. We have created systems which protect us in the aggregate from facing up to the very things that as individuals we most need to know. The surgeon, the hospital, would readily have shielded me from becoming half as involved in Aron's death as I did. It would have been easy to conform to an arbitrarily imposed limit to my responsibility in the matter.

But marriage, even as society understands it, means more than this. Without having gone through an actual wedding ceremony with Aron (and there was really no need ever to have done that) I would have been aware that the responsibility incurred by our relationship had no limit. I had to see him through this thing as far as I conceivably could, or else account to myself for my own cowardice for ever after.

In fact, I needed not to have the burden removed. I needed to face the whole of it, the whole reality of Aron dying, ridiculously young, not having achieved anything he wanted to achieve, knowing there is no God. I had to go every inch of the way with him, to die with him, if I was ever to make anything of life again. Nobody could carry the load for me. Complete involvement was my only hope.

I got to know the disease almost as well as I knew Aron. I recognised the feeling and the smell of it. It was the enemy, but I wasn't afraid anymore, just angry. 'Nothing in life is to be feared,' said Marie Curie. 'It is only to be understood.' Was there perhaps in the back of my mind the wild surmise that somebody who cared as much as I did, might understand cancer enough to find the way to stop it while there was still time? I don't know, but I certainly thought the caring mattered. I regarded the attention that I gave to the disease as a constructive battle. I had a very distinct feeling that I was holding death at bay by looking straight at it.

And as time went on, Aron and the cancer seemed more and more to lead separate existences. I noted every minute change in him. Yet somehow the total effect blurred. I saw Aron apart from the ravages made on his body. I saw his essential being: his gentleness, his courage, his indestructable love of life.

*　　*　　*

The first evening my mother had not yet arrived. I cooked scrambled egg for the three of us. I began to hope very much for an early night. But Aron, now far too tired to eat as much as he did, was almost immediately sick. The nausea persisted for hours. The pain set in. He couldn't swallow the tablets that would have enabled him to settle for the night. I wished I didn't have to cope with this almost the moment he came home. I wished I felt a little less exhausted. I lay down on the studio couch that was to be my bed. All I wanted was rest.

'I can't even see you,' Aron said from the other side of the room after what seemed like only a few minutes. His voice was very small and sad.

'I'm tired,' I pleaded. 'Just let me lie here for a minute.'

There was complete silence. I felt terribly guilty, but I didn't get up.

The doorbell rang. I heard my father going to answer it. He called me from downstairs. I dragged myself to my feet. Danny Cohen had come to ask how Aron was. Danny was a doctor but I had never really thought of him in this capacity. Aron and I knew him and his wife as neighbours, a few years younger than ourselves and exceptionally friendly. It was probably through them that we had been introduced to everybody else we knew in the flats. They were the centre of social life there, and their place was always full of people, all kinds of people. They had no prejudices and a refreshing lack of interest in keeping up appearances of any sort.

During the day, babies and small children sprawled in large numbers about their floor. They were then expecting their own second child. And any infant was welcome there. And any adult who called was invited in for coffee. They also used to lend out all manner of tools and gadgets, so that if the curtain rail fell down or the car battery needed recharging everybody knew where to go for the equipment to put it right. In fact they almost succeeded in turning that urban estate into a kind of village community, where people pulled together a bit and showed a certain concern about each other's problems.

Although I was only slightly acquainted with the Cohens at that time, they were naturally among the first people to whom I took my troubles. They knew all about the illness, but somebody else must have told Danny that Aron had come home because I hadn't had time to tell him that myself yet.

'I don't know if we're going to make it,' I said. 'He's been sick already, and he doesn't want to let me out of his sight for a minute just now.'

'He's tired,' said Danny. 'He'll feel better after a good night's sleep. So will you.'

I wondered if sleep for either of us was at all likely that night.

'Shall I call tomorrow morning?' Danny said, noticing, I suppose, that I wasn't apparently going to invite him in.

'Yes. That would be nice.' I would have liked to ask him upstairs then, but I knew that Aron wouldn't want it. Aron regarded him as a friend, not as a doctor, and he wasn't up to seeing friends without a good deal of warning. He had to screw himself up for it. Since the operation he had only wanted to see even Dylan once.

When I went back to Aron, however, he was obviously reviving. He took his tablets and actually fell asleep. There was to be no crisis after all.

I lay in the darkness with my eyes wide open, listening to his quiet breathing and his every movement. The bedclothes rustled softly when he turned. How exciting it was to have him here! How glad I was that he was home! Whatever happened afterwards, this was wonderful, this one night together in our room again.

I didn't sleep at all, but it hardly mattered. I was so happy. Aron was sleeping soundly. He trusted completely that he would be all right. I felt overwhelmingly protective towards him. I hadn't realised that having him back home could possibly be as good as this.

The moment light begins to break, all the birds get up. For a short time, even in a city, they make a tremendous noise. I think it was something I hadn't known about before that time—the colossal uproar that birds make at daybreak.

In the early hours of the morning my mother arrived. The dawn had been beautiful she said. There was every promise of a glorious day. In spite of the night on the train, she was full of energy, ready to cope with anything.

After breakfast she and my father went out shopping, and Danny came for coffee with Aron and me. I had put on a sleeveless dress that Aron once bought for me to wear at a party. There were no rules anymore. You could wear whatever you liked, and this as much as anything expressed the mood of the day. We talked of trivial things, the sun pouring into the room, the quietness of that first night there. Aron had slept through the awakening of the birds. He told Danny about his illness, the authorised version of it.

'Apparently I'll be ill for a long time,' he said. 'I may even have to go back to hospital.'

'Well, you've only got one liver,' Danny commented gently. 'There's isn't another to keep you going while that one gets better.'

On their way back, my parents met Danny leaving the flat. They asked him how he found Aron.

'Much as I expected really,' he replied.

We all wondered exactly what Danny had expected, whether this was good or bad and what he thought would happen next. We had no idea what sudden turn the illness might take, or even when or how to tell the end was coming. We were ignorant about everything, totally in the dark.

During the weekend Aron got up and sat in a chair in the afternoons. On Sunday we all had tea with him. He was quite unused to talking to more than one person at a time. And when we were still all imagining that he was enjoying himself, he suddenly said, 'I think I'll go to bed.' He was exhausted. We had forgotten how easily overtired he could become. We cleared away the teacups and the extra chairs as quickly and silently as possible.

My mother was leaving on the night train, to return to her kindergarten. She had thought out as many ways as possible of simplifying housekeeping for me during the coming week. The kitchen cupboards and the refrigerator were filled with food that was already prepared or easy to prepare. She was discussing all this with me when it occurred to her that we should carry Aron's record player up to his room before she left.

The record player was very large, with a long, flat, polished lid. I bent over it to lift it up. I remembered the day we first got it. I had disliked it because it was so big, so like a coffin.

But it wasn't like that to Aron. He needed music. He was overjoyed to see it. He had forgotten his tiredness, and sat bolt upright in bed when my mother said goodbye to him. Then he asked for music, more and more music. He chose classical records instead of jazz to please me, because I had no particular enthusiasm for jazz. I didn't want classical records either then. I wanted just to go to bed. I was getting practically no sleep because I had stopped taking my sleeping pills. I was afraid to take them in case they prevented me from hearing Aron in the night. But how could I cut off the pleasure that Aron was taking in this music just because I was tired? It could easily be the last time he would ever enjoy listening to his records. And so Mozart and Beethoven and Bach went on and on. And it was suddenly quite beautiful, the music and this moment. And it didn't matter anymore that I was tired.

At 10.45 p.m. Aron, still buoyant, swallowed two of his tablets. Then he vomited almost immediately. I braced myself. There just wouldn't be any rest for a long time yet. The pain was very bad now, and Aron vomited again.

I heard my father coming back from seeing my mother off on the train. I shouted to him to bring another bowl. I was far calmer than I had been two nights ago. I was quite prepared now to sit up with Aron the whole night if necessary, to sit beside him and take what I could of the pain.

Around midnight, however, he succeeded in swallowing two soluble codeine tablets. He slept soundly until 5 a.m.

In the morning I rang the sister at the hospital and told her that we were all right, that Aron wouldn't be returning there at present, that I would keep him at home.

'I'm very glad to hear this,' she said. 'I'll tell Mr. Warfield-Scrogge as soon as I see him. It will be the first thing he asks.

'You know,' she added, 'I think he'll be surprised. I think he thought you wouldn't manage.'

*   *   *

The only time when it was possible to speak to Dr. Sciberas personally on the telephone was during her surgery hours. The rest of the time, calls were referred elsewhere. I rang her during evening surgery the day that Aron came home. I told her that Aron would be at home for the weekend or possibly longer, and that I would be grateful if she could look in and see him. She sounded affable, but didn't come to see us during the weekend.

She had also given the impression over the phone that she still knew practically nothing about the case, and this troubled me a bit. During our last week in hospital Dr. Lewis had been replaced by another house surgeon, but I understood that the new doctor was phoning Dr. Sciberas the day that Aron came home. I also thought that reports had been sent earlier to Dr. Sciberas. In fact, I never discovered the extent of the communication, if any, that had taken place up to this point, because Dr. Sciberas never at any time admitted to knowing more than a bare diagnosis.

I rang Dr. Sciberas again during her Monday morning surgery, and told her that Aron would be staying on at home. Monday passed, and there was still no visit. This surprised Aron, who had the impression that he was too ill to be out of hospital for long without being seen by a doctor. Why otherwise had Mr. Warfield-Scrogge been so insistent that he should return there at the slightest sign of trouble?

On Monday evening I told Irma that Dr. Sciberas' lack of interest was beginning to upset Aron. Irma said she would do something about it, and in fact rang Dr. Sciberas on Tuesday morning. The result of this was that later on Tuesday Dr. Sciberas rang me. Again she sounded thoroughly affable. She said that I must get in touch with her immediately if anything went wrong.

89

'I'm in a position to get him back into hospital at a moment's notice,' she assured me.

I had never at any time doubted that I was also in that position. But the problem at the moment was not how to get him back to hospital but how to keep him at home, which incidentally was saving the Health Service the whole cost of his upkeep and freeing a bed for somebody who actually needed it. I might have said more about what I was trying to do if I had realised that Dr. Sciberas' phone call was in fact in lieu of a visit. I kept expecting her to turn up at the flat all the rest of Tuesday, but she never came.

On Tuesday evening Irma and Dylan went to Dr. Sciberas' surgery. They got her secretary to put down a visit to Aron as one of the doctor's definite appointments for Wednesday. They also collected all the necessary prescriptions for Aron. They came back quite convinced that Dr. Sciberas would come this time, because they had seen it written in her diary. In my relief, I was stupid enough to tell Aron about the projected visit. I had previously been rather careful not to suggest that any such thing would definitely happen.

Aron got up early on Wednesday. He washed and shaved himself in the bathroom for the first time since he came home. He then got me to help him to organise all the books and records in the room. He had never been so active since the operation. He kept saying how much better he felt, how much better he was sleeping and eating since he came home. Obviously, he was all set to show Dr. Sciberas how beneficial home was.

At 9.25 a.m. he took one of his tablets to set himself up for the morning. I was allocating these very carefully, always giving him soluble codeine instead if it seemed likely to be enough to get him by. He listened to Buddy Tate playing tenor sax in *Let's Jam*. He seemed almost gay.

By noon he was sadder. He said he had a pain, but that codeine would do. He took two codeines dissolved in water. We hadn't mentioned Dr. Sciberas at all. Knowing, however, that her anticipated visit had coloured the whole morning, I remarked as lunchtime approached that she was presumably not coming until the afternoon.

Aron managed some soup and cold chicken for lunch. After it, I began to get the uneasy feeling that, yet again, Dr. Sciberas wasn't coming. I tried to dismiss the whole thing from my mind, but it was difficult to think of anything other than the waiting.

I suppose it was about four o'clock that I abandoned hope. I decided to ring Irma after six. Aron was reading. Perhaps he wasn't particularly concerned, but it seemed unlikely after all the preparations of the morning.

'I can't understand what's happened to Sciberas,' I finally said at six o'clock.

'That's the one thing you do get in hospital,' said Aron, showing that he cared as much as I suspected. 'There are always doctors popping in and out there.'

Irma was shocked to hear that there had been no visit yet, especially as I was becoming a little hysterical about it. She said she would ring Dr. Sciberas at her surgery straight away.

'Where is the street?' Dr. Sciberas said to her. 'I couldn't find it. It's not on the map.'

It was true that our street was too recent to have got on to most maps, but it was hard to imagine that a few inquiries wouldn't have been enough to locate it. The Post Office knew where to bring our letters, and lots of shops had been delivering stuff there for years. Anyway, Dr. Sciberas could have phoned me. She had my number.

Irma told Dr. Sciberas exactly where the street was, and she said she would call after evening surgery.

And so at last she came. Wearing a frilly pink blouse under a smart black suit, she looked immaculately groomed despite her strenuous efforts, which she immediately enlarged upon, to find the place.

'I believe you want to see me,' she said, as if it were with me, rather than Aron, that she was concerned. And she began to walk towards the living room.

91

'Yes, I do. But can we go upstairs first? My husband's longing to see you.'

'I don't know much about him,' she said abruptly.

'You do know what's wrong with him?'

'All I know is that he has cancer of the pancreas. It has affected the liver. Is that correct?'

I nodded. She still hesitated in the hall.

'What will he want to know?' she said.

'Nothing. He doesn't ask any questions.'

Dr. Sciberas looked as if she thought this unlikely. Then she turned sharply and shot upstairs and straight across the bedroom to where Aron lay.

Aron gave every sign of being charmed to see her. She too could be more charming than I'd realised. A very amiable conversation ensued.

'I see you like music,' she said, glancing round the room. And they talked of favourite composers for a few minutes before turning to the more difficult subject of Aron's illness. But there didn't seem to be much difficulty about this either really. She explained that Aron would be short of a particular vitamin that is normally stored in the liver, and that she would prescribe a pleasant-tasting medicine to replace this.

In fact, the medicine, called Cytacon, was a huge success with Aron. So was the whole visit, although he wondered why she had seen no need to examine him. As she was going downstairs Dr. Sciberas remarked, within Aron's hearing, that she would look in again soon. Then, alone with me, her tone changed completely.

'Now,' she said rather grimly as we walked into the living room, 'what exactly do you want me to do for you?'

'I want you to help me to keep him at home,' I said at once. 'I don't want him to go back to hospital.'

She shrugged.

'This is very brave and all that,' she said. 'But it won't work, you know.'

I stood and waited for her to explain why. We were both

standing because she looked as if she hadn't time to sit down.

'The pain is easy,' she said. 'We can always deal with pain. It's the one thing we are equipped to cope with. We always have someone who can be called in quickly to give an injection. We never let a patient go on suffering pain.'

I was very relieved to hear this, because it was the pain that worried me most. I was afraid of Aron suffering because I couldn't get him an injection as quickly as the hospital. But Dr. Sciberas hadn't finished.

'It's all the other things that we can't manage,' she said. 'Incontinence of urine and faeces, incessant vomiting, vomiting of blood—things like that become impossible to manage at home. Hospital facilities are essential.

'Then there's the danger of you becoming so absolutely worn out with it that he sees you've had enough. When that happens he probably won't want to be a burden to you any longer. He'll hate what you have to put up with. It will be kinder to let him go to hospital.'

I gaped at her in horror.

'It needn't be like this, need it? I mean, the ward sister didn't seem to think that anything like this would happen. She thought he would just get weaker and weaker, and that I would probably be able to look after him myself most of the time . . .' My voice dwindled to a whisper under her expression.

'Oh dear me, no!' she said, raising the line of her neatly plucked eyebrows. 'That's not it at all. If he stays here for any time, he's almost bound to have to go into hospital occasionally anyway—for stomach wash-outs and so forth. It's a very wearing business, that. I've seen patients become so tired of being shunted backwards and forwards to hospital, that in the end they just want to stay there. You can see it in their eyes. They're in such a frightful condition that they don't want their wives to be subjected to it anymore.'

I saw Aron with sad, tired, pleading eyes, being carried out of the flat. His plea was that I wouldn't try to keep him with me any longer. I was to regard him as simply the wreckage of his former self. I was to let him die, away from me, in a place where they knew how to cope with the total disintegration of a human being.

I was extremely frightened, but I still knew it wasn't true. Somehow, despite her superior knowledge, what Dr. Sciberas was saying wasn't true. The thing between Aron and me could never be destroyed like this. There would never be a time when he would choose the hospital instead of me.

Before she left, the doctor assured me yet again that she could get Aron back to hospital at a moment's notice. I think she wanted to emphasise her influence there, but a new fear began to form in my mind. Supposing she tried to do this, in spite of me, in spite of my desire to go on nursing my husband at home. She had more authority than I. She was in a stronger position altogether, and as far as I could see she wasn't on my side.

Moreover, I was badly shaken by her description of the horrors to come. It was at least as alarming as anything that Mr. Warfield-Scrogge had said, and some of the details were new ideas to me. It might be simply ghastly at the end. I'd just have to face that, if and when it happened.

Aron at least was glad that Dr. Sciberas had finally made it. Aron had enjoyed the visit.

8

The challenge presented by Aron's homecoming carried me through every obstacle at first, but after about a week I began to wonder how long I could go on without more sleep than I was getting. Although this was a situation in which it was practically impossible to sleep without pills, I continued not to take them in case they knocked me out too much to be of any use to Aron in the night.

Had Dr. Sciberas been different, I would have asked her what to do about this. But she was what she was and if told, I thought, would very likely cite it as yet another reason for giving in. Nursing Aron for twenty-four hours a day was theoretically impossible; a day consists of approximately three nursing shifts. The ward sister, however, had apparently thought it possible, so I rang her to see what would happen if I took my sleeping pills.

She asked what the pills were, then said immediately, 'Oh, those won't knock you out. Those are just to settle your nerves. You should take them. I think you really need them.'

I slept a lot more after that, but the odd thing was that I never missed anything that happened to Aron. I think there was no need for him even to make a sound in order to attract my attention. As soon as he wakened I was awake too. Awake or asleep we were in constant communication.

As well as collecting all Aron's prescriptions and finally prevailing upon Dr. Sciberas to come, Irma and Dylan had arranged for the district nurse to pay us weekly visits. They had fixed this up with Dr. Sciberas' secretary, whom I never met but who seemed to be a most efficient and helpful person.

Sometime during the following week the nurse paid her first call. Her name was Mrs. Polly, and she came riding on her bicycle. A sturdy Italian woman, who somehow coped with seven children as well as her job, she obviously knew how to take life as it came. She must have spent a minimal amount of time on her appearance. She didn't bother with make-up, for instance. And her black, wavy hair was just crammed anyhow under her nurse's cap. But there was about her a kind of contentment that made a greater impact than mere looks. Happiness is in itself attractive.

'I am so glad to have a young patient,' she said when she saw Aron. She spoke very correct English with a slight Italian accent. 'Most of my patients are so old, you know.'

Then she took off her coat and rolled up the sleeves of her uniform as far as her plump elbows. While she was giving Aron a blanket bath, she talked all the time about her children and her husband who taught classics, but she never paused in her work. She was quick and gentle, good to have around. From the first, I saw her as a definite lifeline when things got really difficult. But Aron, I think, had no particular feelings about her at that time. For one thing, he was longing to have a proper bath. It was one of the first things he said after he came home, 'Now I can have a proper bath.' But he wasn't strong enough. He was never strong enough again. The bath was always being postponed until tomorrow.

When she had finished, I accompanied Mrs. Polly downstairs and she gave me her telephone number with instructions not to hesitate to use it if I needed her for anything.

'He is very nice,' she said, 'and so cheerful.'

She smiled so much that I began to wonder if she actually knew the prognosis.

'You know what's wrong with him?' I said, the usual tears

threatening at the mere mention of the subject. It was such a bore, this tendency to cry whenever I wasn't with Aron.

'Yes, dear,' she said, looking as if some providence ought to have spared her the necessity of admitting it.

'Still . . .' she added. 'He has you . . . He is very happy.'

As she rode off on her bicycle, which was the latest type of very small machine and practically invisible beneath her, the music of Jelly Roll Morton was sounding loudly from upstairs. A good sign this: Aron wanted jazz only when he was feeling reasonably well. His collection of jazz records was colossal. Louis Armstrong, Lionel Hampton, Oscar Peterson, Johnny Hodges, Dizzy Gillespie, Sonny Rollins, Buck Clayton, Joe Newman, Duke Ellington, Count Basie, Stan Getz—those and many other names had become familiar to me without my particularly listening to their music. But now jazz meant so much to Aron that I began almost to like it too: jazz, the sound of surprise, the careless throwaway thing that achieves lucidity without apparently trying. Out of improvisation—suddenly 'soul'.

All his senses were heightened in those days and, I suppose, disturbed. He was acutely sensitive to smells and tastes as well as sounds. But the same perfume that delighted him one day might very easily revolt him the next. He became fascinated by flowers, as if he had never really looked at one before. And shapes and colours sometimes excited him enormously. I remember him becoming almost ecstatic about the crystal glasses, crushed ice cubes and grapevine colours in an advertisement for some cocktail or other. Perhaps it was a compensatory side-effect of the illness—this increased capacity of his for finding beauty and stimulation everywhere.

* * *

My mother decided to give up her job for the time being, and come and help us. She was devoted to her kindergarten, but this was a sacrifice that I accepted without demur, indeed had been expecting her to make for some time now. I thought the whole world should be eager to revolve round Aron and me, and I wanted my mother to come rather than Aron's mother because this would mean making fewer adjustments myself. My mother would run things my way. There would be a great deal that we needn't explain or discuss.

So my mother came and shouldered all the domestic responsibilities leaving me free to concentrate entirely on nursing Aron. She brought the car with her and, from then on, produced anything that Aron wanted, from a slice of chicken to a fresh pineapple, at a moment's notice.

It was now about ten days after Dr. Sciberas' visit, and she hadn't come again. I knew that Aron was always hoping that she would appear. The district nurse was nice but not sufficiently qualified in medical matters to give him the feeling that he was getting proper, scientific attention. The thing became a mounting worry in my mind. Then, Irma who called to see me frequently, mentioned that Dr. Sciberas had explained the position to her. Apparently the doctor had decided not to visit Aron for psychological reasons. She thought that, with cases of this kind, it was depressing for the patient if the doctor visited often.

I could hardly believe my ears. If Dr. Sciberas thought this, why had she not told me? What she had in fact said to me, and Aron, was that she would come again soon. Did she not believe that Aron would take this literally? Did she really not believe that he wanted to see her?

Ten more days elapsed without sight or sound of her. And little things that happened in the meantime tended to aggravate the feeling of neglect her absence gave me. For instance, one day a pleasant lady in a uniform called at the flat.

'I'm the health visitor,' she said, and for a moment I thought that somebody had come at last without actually being solicited. We had to ask for everything we got. We might never have got the services of the district nurse, had Irma not known how to request it. It would be so nice to get some evidence that the hospital hadn't written us off completely.

98

But it turned out that the health visitor had come to the wrong door. She was really looking for Jenny, who had almost that minute come out of hospital with her new baby. Apparently it was only for healthy babies that such services were automatically laid on.

Another day a doctor called at the flat. He announced himself as Doctor Somebody-or-other, and then he said that he was canvassing for the Liberal party. It amazed me that a doctor had time to do any such thing. Maybe Dr. Sciberas was out canvassing for some cause or other, and that was why she never came. Or perhaps she was the only doctor who really had no time to spare. Perhaps we were as unlucky as that.

One morning it all got too much for me, and I burst into tears over the breakfast table. I usually had breakfast downstairs with my parents.

'If only we had a normal doctor,' I sobbed. 'It's not much to ask, just a doctor who would come and see us and behave normally.'

My father decided to confront her, and set off soon afterwards for morning surgery. As it turned out, it was Dr. Sciberas' partner Dr. Sidebotham, who was taking the surgery that day. Dr. Sidebotham was an asthmatic, elderly gentleman, with rimless bifocal spectacles and a slight limp. He was very civil and sympathetic with my father, and as far as I could make out their conversation was rich in old-world courtesies. But my father did in fact come straight to the point.

'We want to know if Dr. Sciberas intends to visit,' he said, 'because if not we shall have to try to find somebody who will.'

'Oh tut, tut, dear me, no, you mustn't do that!' said Dr. Sidebotham. 'Oh no, no, no, no! Dr. Sciberas will visit him.'

He went on to explain how busy they had both been lately, and that he himself had just recovered from an illness. He said that Aron was really his patient, and that this was the explanation for the apparent neglect. He produced a folder about Aron, which I was glad to hear existed, and promised to pay a weekly visit himself thereafter. Dr. Sciberas would also call from time to time, he said.

Sidebotham also asked my father how Aron was, what sort of colour he looked, how he was eating. My father couldn't answer these questions in any detail, because he was seeing so little of Aron these days. It was one of the features of the illness, that Aron hardly ever felt up to seeing even the people he most liked. Dr. Sidebotham said he would call at the flat after surgery, and in fact came.

He was almost as much of a success with Aron as Dr. Sciberas had been. He even examined him, which Aron found reassuring. What Aron wanted was to feel that he was being looked after by somebody who understood his condition and would do everything possible to remedy it. This seemed to me a natural thing to want, but neither of the two general practitioners ever seemed to see it that way. Between them they produced all manner of devious arguments to suggest that the ordinary, normal attitude couldn't possibly apply to a patient in Aron's position. Even when he was paying us regular visits Dr. Sidebotham continued to do this. I think he never ceased to believe that it was I, not Aron, who wanted him there. In fact, his visit went splendidly until he came downstairs. Then the thing to which I was growing accustomed happened.

In the most melancholy tones, the doctor proceeded to tell the family group how desperately serious the situation was.

'He's very ill,' he said as if we hadn't realised that he was dying of cancer. 'Very ill indeed.'

I noticed my father bending a little towards him in his anxiety, being affected by the statement in much the way that I had been affected by earlier statements of Dr. Sciberas and Mr. Warfield-Scrogge. I'd had enough of it. I could assess the gravity of the situation better than Dr. Sidebotham who hadn't seen Aron until today. Aron had been very ill indeed when he came home.

'Shsh!' I said, pointing at the ceiling. The doctor was standing almost immediately below the spot where Aron's bed was in the room above, and he was talking moderately loudly.

'It's all right. He can't hear us here,' said my father a little angrily. He may have realised that what I felt was intolerance towards the doctor rather than alarm at the possibility of Aron overhearing us.

'The carcinoma has spread to most of the structures in the abdomen. The liver is badly affected,' Sidebotham continued, in a hushed whisper now.

There was a frightened silence.

'How long would you say he will last?' said my father.

'Not more than about three weeks,' said the doctor.

That meant until about the end of November, I thought. But Aron had already gone past two of Mr. Warfield-Scrogge's deadlines. The end of October was the longest the surgeon ever anticipated for him. I looked away. I was just sick of it. I didn't believe anything that any of them said anymore.

'Are you sure you don't want me to arrange for him to go back to hospital?' said Sidebotham. 'I know you probably don't want to suggest it to him, and it would be easier perhaps if it came from me.'

Everybody looked at me.

'No,' I said.

'She's very determined,' said my father.

I would have liked to explain how much home meant to Aron, but I couldn't trust myself to do it without bursting into tears. And that would give Dr. Sidebotham quite the wrong impression as well as a very distinct advantage. I mustn't let him think that there was any weakness in me anywhere.

'You feel that if he left here, he would look at you more in sorrow than in anger,' said the doctor. 'Well, I can understand that. Well, we'll just have to see how it goes.'

And so he tottered away, leaving my parents looking pretty sad.

'It's bad what he says about Aron,' my father remarked, hunched in a chair, the light shining on his white hair.

'It doesn't mean very much, does it?' I retorted. 'After all, nobody knows that he's any worse than he was when he first came home. It's more than three weeks since then, and this is the first time that any doctor has examined him here.'

'Yes, but Sidebotham seems nice,' my mother said soothingly. 'He'll come and visit him now.'

I hoped so, but I also hoped that next time he would take more interest in the amount of sedation I was giving Aron. I was disappointed that he had simply written out the usual re-peat prescriptions, and shown no interest in what Aron and I were actually achieving. This was very little different from ringing the secretary at the surgery and getting the prescriptions posted or left in a box to be collected. With the help of a doctor who took a real interest in the detail, I thought it might be possible to improve on the delicate balance that was keeping Aron alive.

I was completely absorbed in this business of administering Aron's drugs to the best possible advantage. I noted down every tablet that I gave him, together with the precise time it was given, and I observed his reactions minutely. Oddly, perhaps, my record of all this became neater and tidier as time went on.

The immediate effect of bringing Aron home had been to cut down his intake of palfium tablets by half. For the first three weeks at home, he took on average three tablets a day instead of the six he had been having in hospital. For a further two weeks he rarely exceeded four tablets a day. Instead of the other tablets he took soluble codeine and, considering the nausea to which he was frequently subject, it was remarkable how much of this he managed to keep down.

What was it all for? He was going to die in any case, wasn't he? All I can say is that it was in order to stay together as long as possible. Being together was bigger than the illness, more important than anything. And being together was only possible as long as Aron stayed alive.

But of course, his attitude had changed since the beginning of the illness. When he first went into hospital, he seemed almost indifferent as to whether he lived or died. He even said he wanted to die sometimes. Later he never talked like that. It had become plain to everyone that he was fighting for life as hard as he could. I was so much a part of this battle that I think I saw it differently from other people, who felt primarily pity. To me it was worth while in itself, in the way that all heroic gestures are worth while in themselves. People who believe in something don't count the cost. Aron believed in life.

9

Of course there were times when our involvement with each other wasn't enough to blind either of us to the physical facts. The hardest moments were during the relatively short period when Aron noticed what was happening to him. Although it was well into November then, the sunshine continued. But we had to draw the curtains quite a lot, shut out the strong light that hurt his eyes and also perhaps revealed too much.

'Why am I not getting any better?' he said suddenly, angrily, from his chair one afternoon.

'They did say it would take a long time,' I replied.

'But it's no good. I'm not getting any better. Why don't they *do* something?' he exclaimed.

'Because they never do anything,' I said. 'You know that. You know their favourite cure for everything is rest.' I was moving on to safer ground really, for I had always tended to talk of the medical profession like this. I had never shown much faith in the miracles of modern science.

'I wish I could get better,' he said passionately. 'I only wish I could get better.'

I looked at him and there seemed nothing to say. He was yellow and haggard and emaciated. The absence of flesh on his arms and body made his tall frame look even more elongated. His eyes were sunken, and you could see the whole bone structure of his face. I saw all this so accurately at that moment that I wondered how it was possible, so much of the time, not to notice it at all. I never saw it as others saw it, for instance, when I first came into the room. However briefly we were parted, each reunion was somehow so marvellous that it blinded me to everything else. In fact I think it was only because Aron had drawn attention to it that I saw clearly what the disease was doing to him even then. I noticed it only when he did. My mood, my state of mind, depended absolutely on his.

'What is the matter with me?' he said.

'Do you really want to know?' I replied before I had time to register that this was it. This was the question I had once been dreading daily but finally ceased altogether to expect. Now I had virtually given the show away. God, I was useless! Why had I not thought first and spoken afterwards?

'To know exactly, I mean,' I added hastily.

But Aron had either taken warning, or been genuinely unaware of the implications of my question. I never knew which. He shrugged and looked away.

'Not really,' he said, as if he thought the details would only bore him.

'Would you like to hear a record?'

'Yes, all right,' he agreed with a quick, brave smile that didn't deceive me.

While the Elgar was playing I sat and wondered how I should have answered his question. After all, he had a right to the truth if he wanted it. Perhaps he ought to know it, if he didn't know it already. He would face it far better than I did. I was certainly afraid of having it openly acknowledged between us. I felt that this would be a situation far too painful to live with. And perhaps Aron knew all this. Dr. Sidebotham contended that he did. Dr. Sidebotham said that Aron knew, but wanted to protect me from the knowledge. Perhaps this wasn't as far-fetched as I thought it at the time.

Anyway, I was angry with myself for having coped with the situation so badly, but I was angry about nearly everything at that time. I suppose I had reason to be depressed, but depression happens independently in any case. It occurs not necessarily

105

for any reason other than the fact of sitting around too much and moping, being shut off from outside stimuli. Any number of things might have made me snap out of it, regain my former attitude about the value of what I was doing. Maybe it would only have taken something like a visit from Clive.

Aron's reluctance to see anybody but me had increased of late. I suppose it was becoming more and more difficult for him to live up to his own image of his former self. He knew he had changed, and the effort of pretending otherwise took more out of him than he had to spare. For some time Danny had been the only visitor from outside who was automatically admitted to Aron's room. Then Danny went away on holiday, and when he came back Aron said he wasn't feeling up to seeing him that day. The next day it was the same. Fearing that Aron might never feel up to seeing Danny again, I took matters into my own hands and invited him upstairs nonetheless.

I did this because Danny was a doctor, and from then on I think that Aron regarded him rather more as a doctor too. But of course apart from the reassurance of having somebody with his professional qualifications around, I benefitted enormously from his visits myself. Particularly during this black period, I missed the contact with friends of my own age and way of thinking. I loved Irma's visits. I wished that other people would phone and call to see me, whether or not Aron was well enough to be visited. I wanted to feel that I was still part of the world in which Aron and I had previously moved.

Hardly any of our friends seemed to realise this. Most of them waited, in silence, at a safe distance, for the thing to end. Clive would ring at longish intervals, mainly to see whether it was over or not, I felt. Latterly he took to ringing other people, like Dylan, for this information. Communication with my former colleagues virtually ceased. I tried to ring my editor once but he wasn't there. I left a message for him to ring me back, but he never rang.

One day Dylan accidentally bumped into a college friend of his and Aron's, who had since become a university teacher.

Apparently, on hearing about Aron, this friend turned deathly pale and scurried away looking as if he might easily step out in front of the first passing bus. Maybe he did, because I never heard from him at all again. Strange that these people who spent so much of their time thinking and sorting out ideas, should have felt that they had nothing to contribute to a situation like ours! Until then I had always regarded intellectuals as people who tried to penetrate rather than escape from life.

But then of course my attitude to Aron's parents was part of the same thing. Something separated me from them—something that surely ought to have had the opposite effect. Life had given me more than it had given them, and I should have been able to use this in some way that helped. Instead I found communication increasingly difficult. I dreaded their phone calls when I had to speak for Aron, try to tell them the sort of things he'd tell them.

I was really a mass of contradictions, wanting my own parents to be there, for instance, and yet at that time also feeling inhibited by their presence. I think I fancied that if they weren't around, it might be possible to recapture something of what it had been like before, alone with Aron in the flat. I suppose I resented being as dependent on them as I was. As always they understood, and they began to go out quite often for a considerable part of the day.

Displays of temperament from me were fairly common then, but however much I took out my resentment on other people, I couldn't stop Aron from noticing the ghastly physical deterioration that was going on. I remember him standing in the bathroom one morning, looking at the way his stomach had swollen out around the disappearing scar.

'I look like something out of Belsen,' he said. 'Oh, the filth! The filth inside me!'

The nights were the worst. Evening after evening, Aron had such difficulty in swallowing the tablet that might have given him some rest. The hour that he attempted to do this varied according to the pattern of the rest of the day. It had to be before the effect of the previous tablet had completely worn off. Otherwise, he was too tired to keep it down. But whatever time he tried to take it, he was likely to vomit the thing up again at the first attempt. After that, the difficulty of taking another was enormously increased. Usually he had to wait for an hour or so before even trying again. During that time he became more racked and worn out than ever, less likely to be able to absorb the drug.

Occasionally, out of sheer exhaustion, he fell asleep without it, or with a couple of codeine instead. But when that happened, he usually woke up to repeat the whole performance later. At 2 or 3 or 4 a.m. he would again be trying to swallow the thing and again be vomiting it up.

'Sometimes I think I'm dying,' he said on one such occasion. 'Have you been in touch with the hospital lately?' he added after a moment.

I hadn't. At first, I used to phone the sister every now and then. But I found the last conversation with her so embarrassing that I hadn't rung again. The trouble was that she got on to the subject of religion.

'It's the only consolation,' she said, and then she described the progress of the other similar patient in the ward, the one who didn't have a private room and whose wife visited him in the surroundings that I found so deplorable. Apparently this man knew that he was dying, but he refused to accept it. He just kept fighting. According to the sister this was a dreadful thing for his wife to have to watch. On her advice, the man's wife had sought the help of the hospital chaplain, who had converted the patient. It was the answer, the only answer, according to the sister. The man accepted his death now. He was resigned, at peace. She proceeded to question me quite seriously about the possibility of bringing the same solace to Aron.

Perhaps for this other man, it was the answer. Perhaps it was always in him to be religious, and all his life was pointing towards the ultimate discovery of God. But that wasn't like

Aron. I couldn't possibly have told her how much the idea horrified me as applied to Aron, what a sickening betrayal of his real self it seemed. Memories of his Marxist days at Oxford, admiration for his clear, uncluttered, rational view of life, cried out in his defence. He was weak, exhausted. He relied on me. Maybe I could have persuaded him to listen to religion, although I doubt it. But what a breach of my allegiance it would have been! What abuse of power! This was not the time to alter his opinion of anything. The one thing I could do was help him to die as he had lived.

Actually, in spite of the persistent linking of religion with dedicated nursing, a key publication prepared for the International Council of Nurses, reflects my attitude absolutely. 'The unique function of the nurse,' it says, 'is to assist the individual, sick or well, in the performance of those activities contributing to health or its recovery (or to peaceful death) that he would perform unaided if he had the necessary strength, will or knowledge.' The nurse assists her patient, it explains, by contributing to 'what is—to him—a good death.'

In any case, Aron was unhappy and in pain but he wasn't afraid. Lying in the same room with him, night after night, listening to his quiet breathing, wakening at his slightest movement, I would have known at once if he had been afraid.

What he needed much more than religion was an analgesic that he could absorb more easily than those tablets. He ought to be getting injections at night now, when he found it impossible to swallow the pills. But Dr. Sidebotham seemed to regard this as too drastic a step to take yet. It made no sense really, for if Aron had still been in hospital Mr. Warfield-Scrogge would certainly have had him heavily sedated with morphia long before this. Anyway, I felt that when the system was providing so little in the way of practical relief from pain, it added insult to injury to start touting the opiate of religion.

He would get injections if he went back to hospital, of course. I think we both knew this. Was that why he had asked about the hospital?

109

'I haven't been in touch with them for a while,' I told him. 'But you know that you can always go back there any time.'

He thought he was going to be sick. He was sitting with his feet over the edge of the bed, and I was holding him tightly, supporting his back with my arm.

'I don't want to go back to that place,' he said with some vehemence.

So there it was, his decision, made at a time when he could scarcely have been feeling worse. I would never let them take him away after that. Still, it wasn't enough, just then, being at home. It was a bad time. Yet, due to the urgency of Dr. Sidebotham's pessimism, it was precisely at that time that Aron's parents were asked to come and see their son again.

When they came, they stayed with Irma and Dylan because there wasn't any more room in the flat. But of course they spent all day with us. Aron was pleased to hear they had arrived, but added that he would see them later. He said this every time the subject came up, all day. Perhaps he was afraid of being unable to blind himself to their reaction to his appearance. Perhaps he just wanted to work up all the energy he had for the occasion. Anyway, I thought it better not to force a meeting. I kept waiting for Aron to take the initiative until, in the early evening, his father understandably lost patience and burst into the room. He must have got a dreadful shock.

Aron was sitting propped up in a chair, looking like living death. For anyone who hadn't seen him for several weeks, there could no longer be any possibility of doubt about what the end would be. Had I had time to set the scene, I would certainly have arranged that Aron was in bed. He looked much better in bed, more relaxed and less obviously emaciated. Also he had more energy to spare when he was lying down. But this was how it happened. And I just shut myself off from it, tried not to think about it at all.

I have vague memories of Aron's mother coming smiling to his bedside and presenting him with sponge cakes; of the two parents sitting there remembering the baby and the boy who was so good at cricket and always top of the class, trying to make last connections that would remain with them for the rest of their lives. But I simply couldn't contemplate the details of this final interlude, and have forgotten most of them. I hardly discussed anything with Aron's parents. I left this to my parents who did all the talking, all the comforting.

During the day there seemed to be so much talking, and I had grown accustomed to long silences, especially in the afternoons. It was better when I didn't join the others downstairs. I was so critical so much of the time, drawing attention, for instance, to things that were in the wrong place because Aron's mother had put them there in her desire to help. I would become idiotically upset if I found the kitchen cutlery mixed up with the rest, or failed to find something quite unimportant like my usual napkin ring.

But when the day came for Aron's parents to go, the mixture of emotions was even worse. They were so matter-of-fact; a better word for it is brave. Aron must have got his courage from them. This time there was no reassurance from me that they would ever see him alive again. The chances were that he would be unconscious if they did. But they said goodbye to him in much the way they must have done when they left him, as an eight-year-old evacuee, with his grandparents in the Rhondda Valley. I wasn't with them when they said goodbye of course. I always left them to talk to Aron by themselves. But there were no tears, no scenes. And his mother came downstairs saying that he was feeling a good deal better.

'He told me that I must get a taxi from the station,' she said. 'He made me promise to get a taxi.'

And so they went away. And it was true, Aron was much better. Something, perhaps the need to help his parents, had enabled him to stop caring about his own condition at all. Physically, nothing had changed, but Aron himself was suddenly at peace. If he had been converted to religion by then, the thing would certainly have been attributed to God, for the virtues that he displayed were essentially Christian ones.

There he lay, crucified, his long hair matted on the pillow, and all his sympathy was for those around him, not for himself. Everything he said was kind and full of gentleness: 'You must be tired of this. It's awful for you.' He was suddenly much more aware of the other lives revolving round him, thanked my mother for everything she was doing, asked to see my father who had almost despaired, I think, of ever being wanted in his room again. This attitude persisted from that day until the end.

10

Now the air was cold and crisp outside The last leaves had finally fallen, and it began to seem like winter. There was a sparrow that often sat huddled on the window sill, almost leaning against the pane. We put out water and breadcrumbs and bits of bacon rind for it, and all the other birds started to come too, chirping loudly and squabbling with each other and splashing water from the metal dish. Aron would sometimes stand and watch them, amused and interested. In the daytime he could still push aside the illness for quite long periods. But at night the pain was getting out of hand. Even if he managed to swallow them, his little white pills no longer necessarily helped. We needed something better.

On two successive nights I rang for a doctor in the middle of the night. As always when ringing Dr. Sciberas' number outside surgery hours the calls were automatically referred to a telephone answering service. This organisation asked first of all for the name of the patient and the address. (I always had to go into some detail about the address, knowing that our street wasn't on the map and feeling that this provided any doctor with a good excuse for failing to arrive.) They then asked the age of the patient and the diagnosis (a thing I hated to discuss). After that they inquired into the reasons for wanting a doctor at that particular time. In fact, the conversation went on for ages. A better system for deterring calls from relatives of people dying of cancer could scarcely have been devised.

The first night I did this, the telephone answering service told me that a doctor would come in about an hour. One did. He was a pleasant, athletic young man, who appeared not to have been told anything of the diagnosis I had already provided. Before he bounded up to the bedroom, I had to give him the whole story again. There seemed to be very little that it was actually within his power to do. There was never any question of giving Aron an injection. It wasn't part of the treatment prescribed for him at that stage.

But the young doctor had patience and a certain authority. In his congenial company, Aron succeeded in swallowing two of his usual tablets.

The second night, an Indian doctor came. He muttered apologetically that he knew nothing about the patient. I launched into the grim details for the fourth time in two nights.

The Indian doctor put his large black bag on the floor beside Aron's bed, and asked some routine questions. He opened the bag and peered into it, for all the world like some genie about to produce the panacea. To my astonishment, what he produced was a large bottle of medicine. He poured some into Aron's drinking glass and, by some extraordinary fluke, Aron, who had been vomiting off and on for hours, gulped it all straight down.

'That will put you to sleep,' the doctor said, and took his leave. I think we would both have liked him to stay a little longer, because our faith in the potion was only slight. In fact, the medicine had no effect at all. It was several hours more before either of us got any rest.

A few days later, because of the persistent pain, my mother rang for the doctor in the early morning. She was told that Dr. Sciberas herself would come before morning surgery. She and my father went out shopping because they knew I wanted to tackle Dr. Sciberas myself.

This was the second and last time that Dr. Sciberas visited Aron during the whole of the ten weeks he was at home. She

114

was a person who exuded confidence. Aron had far more faith in her than in the kindlier Dr. Sidebotham. She could have done so much for him, had she only seen, or wanted to see, that it was there for her to do.

I don't remember much of what happened in the bedroom, except that Aron was overjoyed to see her of course. But I remember very clearly the way she spoke to me as she went out of the front door. She pushed a prescription for pethidine tablets into my hand.

'You understand,' she said, 'that there is really nothing to be done now. The pain has moved into the bone.'

She smiled or grimaced—out of solicitude or sheer embarrassment—I don't know which. Then she rushed off.

I didn't believe that the pain had moved into the bone, and so I hoped that the pethidine tablets might work. My mother got them at once, and Aron had taken one by 10 a.m. Half an hour later he took two of his usual pills because the pethidine had made no difference. At two o'clock he tried two pethidine tablets. Again they had no effect, and an hour later he again tried one of his old tablets. This pattern continued all that day and most of the next, which was the day that Dr. Sidebotham paid his regular weekly visit in the evening.

Just before Dr. Sidebotham was due, the pain got worse than it had ever been before. Aron said he couldn't possibly swallow anything without being sick. He lay in one position, as if on a knife edge, not daring to move.

I heard the doorbell ring. I heard Dr. Sidebotham going into the living room for his usual chat with my parents. This time, I thought, he must give Aron an injection. I couldn't just get up and leave Aron because I was part of the battle he was fighting against the pain. I had to prepare him for an absence of even a few minutes.

'I think that Sidebotham has maybe come,' I said, taking care not to sound too positive about it. It might not be Dr. Sidebotham. Aron rarely noticed sounds downstairs now. Either his hearing was duller, or he was too taken up with the struggle inside himself. Contending with the illness was in itself a full-time job.

'Shall I go down and see?' I waited until he nodded his assent. Then I flung myself headlong into the living room.

'Right now,' I announced, 'he has a worse pain than he has ever had before.'

'I'll come straight up,' said the mild-mannered doctor, as I shot away ahead of him upstairs.

Aron looked all flaked out with pain, but he smiled at the sight of the doctor.

'Having a bad patch?' said Sidebotham sympathetically. He bent over Aron to discover where the pain was.

'Take two of your tablets,' he said, stepping back a little. Then he turned to me.

'Give him two of his tablets,' he said with an air of authority.

I held out two pethidine tablets for Aron to take, and Dr. Sidebotham backed away almost to the other side of the room. Aron swallowed the tablets.

'Good!' said Sidebotham, sidling right out of the room. I was terrified that he would leave the flat altogether, because I knew that this could never work. I slipped out after him and whispered urgently, 'Don't go away.'

'I'll be downstairs,' he said.

As soon as I got back to Aron, he vomited up the tablets. At the first opportunity, I went downstairs again. They were all nodding gravely in the living room. I could imagine what Dr. Sidebotham had been saying because he said it every week. It was his regular custom to express surprise at finding Aron still alive, and to point out how much worse he was than he had been the week before.

'You don't see it,' he would say to me, 'because you're with him all the time. But I notice an enormous deterioration over the week.'

I became so immune to this that I used to joke about it after he'd gone. On one occasion poor Dr. Sidebotham was unwise enough to predict only another week for Aron. It was wrong, of course, like his earlier prediction and like both Mr. Warfield-Scrogge's predictions. But now the point was coming when one of these predictions was bound to be right. This was a strange stage in the proceedings to start laughing and playing the fool. Yet that's exactly what I did. I distinctly remember giving the impression of finding Dr. Sidebotham's 'week' very funny indeed.

When I interrupted the gloomy conversation in the living room to announce the failure with the tablets, Dr. Sidebotham adopted an even graver expression than the one he was wearing already.

'I'm afraid I shall have to take a step that I wanted to postpone,' he said. Then he asked for the ampoule of pethidine that he had once left in the flat for an emergency. I was relieved that he was finally taking a decision that seemed to me thoroughly overdue. But I wished it was morphia, not pethidine, that he intended to inject. I knew that morphia worked. I had seen its effect on Aron many times in the hospital. About pethidine, especially after our experience with the tablets, I felt less sure.

'Why don't you give him morphia?' I said with sudden audacity.

'Oh, no, no, no! That won't be necessary. Why do you suggest that?'

'Because he got a lot of it in hospital, and it always worked.'

'What do you mean by a lot?'

'Well, several injections a day for about ten days or a fortnight.'

'Never!' said Sidebotham. 'He might have got it for a day or two after the operation. But ten days . . . Oh, no, no, no, that's not possible.'

'I saw him getting it,' I said.

But Dr. Sidebotham just shook his head. There was no point in arguing. There was too much to explain. Dr. Sidebotham presumably believed that it was always the hospital's intention to let Aron come home. He would never be persuaded that, far from planning this, the initial policy had been to sedate him so heavily that he would be unlikely ever to rise from his bed again.

We went upstairs, and the doctor gave Aron the injection.

'Now you will go to sleep,' he declared. 'Put the lights out,' he told me. Then he tiptoed from the room, leaving a prescription for further ampoules of pethidine on his way out of the flat.

'I'm afraid this is an irrevocable step,' he said despondently.

Everything is irrevocable, I thought returning to the bedroom.

I looked down at Aron in the darkness.

'How do you feel?' I whispered.

'Much the same.'

'It shouldn't be too long before it works,' I said, sitting close beside him.

In fact, it wasn't long. In about half an hour Aron was suddenly, uncontrollably sick. He had never been sick like this before. There was no warning, no time to take any precautions. I had to change all his bed linen.

But the night was only beginning. The terrible pain persisted. At 11.15 p.m. Aron took two pethidine tablets to no avail. At 11.30 p.m. he took two palfium tablets, also to no avail. At about midnight he said, 'This is awful. You'll have to do something.'

'The pain is easy,' I remembered Dr. Sciberas saying what seemed like years ago. 'We can always deal with pain . . . We never let a patient go on suffering pain.'

I went downstairs and dialled the number. The telephone answering service gave me its usual unfriendly grilling. For near-hostile anonymity it certainly took some beating. Even a computer could have stored up some of the information gleaned on previous nights. It said that a doctor would be sent.

I went back upstairs and sat with Aron. Suddenly I realised that the phone was ringing below. It had a very quiet bell. I rushed downstairs again, but by the time I reached it, it had stopped. Assuming that it must have been the telephone answering service, I rang them back. They had in fact been ringing, and had simply given up when they failed to get an immediate reply. They told me to hang on, and then I was put through to somebody who had spoken to Dr. Sciberas.

'She has gone to bed,' I was told, 'and won't be coming.'

'She won't come?' I was incredulous.

'No.'

'Well, why don't you send one of the other doctors?'

'Dr. Sciberas says it isn't necessary. She says that Dr. Sidebotham has already called this evening and given your husband an injection, and that you have an ample supply of tablets. If you can't manage, your husband can go back to hospital.'

'My God!' I said. 'I'll never forget this.'

'Wouldn't he be better back in hospital?' said the girl at the other end, a human being momentarily breaking through the anonymity.

'No,' I said. 'He wouldn't. He doesn't want to go back, and he's not going back. You don't know what it's like there. You don't know the difference it's made to him to be at home. Dr. Sciberas has never been any help, but this is worse than anything. For a doctor to do this . . .'

But words were futile. I had to do something about the pain, and quickly.

'I'll have to find someone else to help,' I said, and put the phone down.

I walked straight out of the flat, dressed as I was in pyjamas and dressing gown. There was still a light on in the Cohen's flat. I rang their bell. In a minute Danny came to the door.

'Aron's got a terrible pain, and Dr. Sciberas has refused to come,' I blurted out at once. 'Have you got anything you could give him?'

'Step inside,' said Danny.

'I've left him alone and he's got this awful pain,' I said, and then I told him as fast as possible everything that had happened that night. 'I'll have to go back,' I added urgently. 'He's got this pain, you see.'

'I'll come round,' said Danny. He seemed to be looking for something in the hall. 'You go on. I'll follow you.'

'Thanks. I'll leave the front door so that you can push it open.'

I ran back to Aron, and told him that Dr. Sciberas wouldn't be coming but that Danny would be with us in a minute. I can't imagine what I would have done if Danny hadn't been coming.

Aron barely reacted to the news. I think he was too far gone with pain. What was it for, this pain? Why Aron? His courage was extraordinary. Why wasn't he complaining? How was he able always to be so gentle with me? He was sitting up against the back of the bed, leaning lightly against me (he must have weighed very little now) when Danny appeared at the door.

'Nobody would know he had a pain,' I said. It was a matter of tremendous pride to be married to somebody as brave as this.

Danny examined Aron very thoroughly, palpating the abdomen with his finger tips. This in itself seemed to help Aron in some way. I noticed that he was relaxing slightly.

'The pain is caused by wind,' said Danny. 'I've tried to move it a little.'

After a while he stood up and regarded us both thoughtfully. He had a calm, intelligent Jewish face, somehow absolutely reliable. He wouldn't ring up the hospital. We were safe with him.

'It will probably go away soon,' he said. 'I tell you what I'll do. I'll leave you now, and come back in an hour or so to see how you're getting on.'

'But that will keep you up most of the night,' I said, knowing quite well he'd never go back on the suggestion once he had made it.

'That's all right. I have reading to do anyway.'

I gave him the key so that he could come straight in without ringing the bell. My parents had slept through everything so far, and this was obviously the best thing in the circumstances.

Before Danny left Aron's pain had diminished and when he

120

came back later it had gone. I don't know whether it was caused by wind or not, but this was a reassuring kind of diagnosis that helped to see us through. Psychology can work sometimes, in the absence of suitable drugs, but it takes more time, more effort, more actual involvement.

11

In the morning I gave my mother a fairly excited account of the night's events. I was excited because I felt that we had scored a victory over Dr. Sciberas, proved anyway that we had the courage of our convictions. We had stuck things out to the point where she had been forced into the open. The situation was clear now. It was no longer a matter of not getting enough support from her. It was a matter of her refusing to look after us at all.

As far as I know, she was quite within her rights. She regarded Aron as a hospital case, and knew that there was always a bed waiting for him there. She had too busy a practice to cope with hospital cases as well. The pity of it was that she hadn't simply told us to find another doctor at the outset. For we too had a right not to be pushed around.

'Or do you think she might try to send Aron back to hospital by force now?' I asked my mother.

'Aron's not going back to hospital,' my mother said. 'There are two of us to contend with now. They'll have to carry him over us both before they get him out of here.'

Aron's helplessness had become a tremendously moving thing. He was so consistently considerate, so sorry if he created work for other people even to the extent of spilling a little orange juice on the bedcover. He was never incontinent, never presented any difficult nursing problems, although I often wondered if this would have been different in hospital. Hospital cancer patients tend to be so much more dramatic, more horrifying. They are primarily cases, not people, and this very possibly affects their physical as well as mental state.

We had quite a succession of visitors that morning. First Danny came, looking very serious indeed but too young to show mere lack of sleep. He had a few words with Aron. Then he drew me aside in the hall.

'Aron's in a very bad state, you know,' he said.

'I know,' I replied.

He nodded. He seemed to believe me at once. He wasn't like the other doctors who thought I hadn't grasped the situation because I could still smile.

'Well,' he said, 'I'll leave a note for Dr. Sidebotham when he comes.'

I wondered whether Dr. Sidebotham would be coming any more. He was, after all, Dr. Sciberas' assistant. However, the note from Danny was obviously a good idea.

The next visitor was Mrs. Polly. She showed very little surprise on hearing of the night's events.

'She will not visit the old people either,' she said. 'This is a bad district for doctors on the National Health. There are many private patients you know . . . But Dr. Sciberas, she is a hard woman, very ambitious . . . I do not know what happened to her husband,' she added irrelevantly.

'Her husband?'

'Yes, she was married. She has a child—well, he is about twenty-five now. I think they separated soon after he was born. Her husband was a doctor too, very clever. They were both very clever. She wanted to become a surgeon, but had to give it up because of the child. She had to bring him up on her own. That was why she went into general practice.'

'She might have made a better surgeon,' I said.

'Yes. I think she was always bitter about it. There are not so many women surgeons, and she was a brilliant student.'

'But it was her own decision—I mean, having the child.'

'Well, some people think it is their duty.'

123

'But she didn't, did she?'

The nurse smiled.

'It is not for me to know that,' she said. 'She is a woman who very much wanted always to have everything perhaps—a husband, a family, a career.'

'Do you think she will try to send Aron back to hospital now?'

'She cannot do that. He is all right here. We can look after him. He is no trouble. He is the sort of patient who must be at home.'

But he needs injections. What will happen about injections?'

'I can give injections. Once he is written up for this, the nurses can do it. He must not go back to hospital,' she said.

Later in the morning, Dr. Sidebotham came, but I didn't know about this until afterwards. I was with Aron, and the doctor didn't come upstairs or ask for me. He always preferred to talk to my parents actually. Perhaps it was because my father had got him to come in the first place. Perhaps it was because they were more nearly the same generation, had more in common altogether. Anyway, he had never called unexpectedly like this before, and the visit was obviously as a result of hearing what had happened the previous night. He spent some time, not exactly apologising, but explaining to my parents how very overworked Dr. Sciberas was. He read Danny's note and said he was tremendously grateful to our neighbour, and would write and thank him for his kindness.

If I had seen him I would have mentioned the effect of the injection as I saw it, but I wouldn't have expected this to make him alter his opinion about pethidine. After all, he knew what a panic there had been later the same night, and he didn't suggest prescribing a different analgesic himself. I thought I would be in a better position to discuss this if I knew exactly what injections Aron had been given in hospital. So I rang up the ward.

Most of the ward staff who knew Aron had been moved elsewhere. The sister, who seemed a fairly permanent fixture, was off duty. While I was waiting for them to find somebody who knew about Aron's treatment, I thought how traumatic it would be for him if he ever did go back now. His little room would almost certainly be occupied by someone else. All the familiar faces would be gone. All the benefits of growing accustomed to the place completely lost. It would be like starting from scratch again, all frightened and anonymous and alone.

I was put through to the house surgeon who had replaced Dr. Lewis. I told him our doctor wouldn't believe the amount of morphia Aron had been getting in hospital, and asked him precisely what the doses were.

He said it would take some time to look up the records.

I told him what had happened after the pethidine injection.

'It would have been the same if he'd had morphia,' he said at once. 'We regard morphia and pethidine as more or less interchangeable. If your doctor gave him pethidine, that was as likely to help as anything else. There's no need to worry on that score.'

I knew even then that this wasn't really true, but doctors always stick together. I should have asked the question another way.

I told him about the system that operated if I rang for a doctor at night; how I had to provide the diagnosis each time; how nobody could give Aron an injection because there were no written instructions to that effect. He offered to send me a note describing the hospital's diagnosis and treatment. The note came some ten days or a fortnight later. We had solved the problem by then.

I wound up by saying how happy Aron was at home, and how important it was that he should stay there.

'That's all very well,' he replied. 'But you must look after yourself you know. You must do this only as long as your own health stands up to it.'

I wished I hadn't raised the subject. He had obviously no idea what I was talking about.

I think it was a day or two later that Danny said: 'You know I expected Aron to be back in hospital by now.'

'Even you!'

'What do you want to do?' he asked me.

'I want to see it through . . . to the end.'

'All right,' he said after a moment. 'All right, I'll help you.'

From then on there were no more worries about doctors. Danny provided the moral support that Aron needed from the medical profession.

But the problem about analgesics continued. The pethidine tablets never helped. Danny sat with Aron for hours on Saturday, administering them at intervals and observing their non-effect. There were of course the ampoules of pethidine that Dr. Sidebotham had prescribed. Aron knew about these, and at the end of that day he asked Danny if he would give him an injection.

'You want me to give you an injection?' Danny repeated before he proceeded with it. But after it the pain redoubled and nausea set in. I was convinced now that pethidine disagreed with Aron. I determined that he shouldn't be given any more, ever.

My mother went to see Dr. Sidebotham and explain this. She asked him if he would prescribe something else. I felt that he would believe her more readily than he would believe me. Even so, he was apparently extremely sceptical about the whole theory until she mentioned that his own injection had made Aron sick.

'My injection!' he exclaimed. 'My injection made him sick!'

Dr. Sidebotham was actually extremely good at giving injections. Aron commented on the fact, then and later. Of course it wasn't the way he gave it; it was the drug itself that was at fault. Fortunately, he began to accept this as a possibility, and wrote out a prescription for morphia. He handed this to my mother with many warnings and intimidations. But he also arranged for the district nurse to give Aron an injection each evening to make him sleep.

There followed another of Dr. Sidebotham's frequent conversations about the pointlessness of his own visits. He persistently refused to believe that Aron really wanted to see him or that his presence did any good. And yet, analgesics apart, he prescribed all kinds of effective antidotes to the unpleasant minor symptoms of the disease: anti-emetics, medicine to avert hiccoughs, soothing mouthwashes and lozenges. He was never stuck for ideas, and nothing he prescribed was useless.

After we got the morphia, I asked Danny to show me how to give injections, because I knew that I might have to do it myself. There would be times when there weren't any doctors or nurses around, and we couldn't always be calling Danny.

He gave me a demonstration, laughing at me a little because he saw that I was squeamish about it. Actually, I hated the thought of giving Aron an injection. I was the sort of person who felt peculiar at the idea of sticking needles into people at all—a physical coward, I think. I couldn't have suffered pain uncomplainingly as Aron did. He had a kind of courage I have never had.

My mother knew all this, and when Danny left she volunteered to give the injections instead of me. She hadn't done it before either, but had no particular reluctance to begin. From the first she was confident about it, and good at it.

*   *   *

The morphia made an enormous difference. At first it did more than dull the pain. It worked on Aron like a tonic. He seemed far better in every way. After its introduction there was another period of great happiness, similar to the one when he first came home. It included his birthday, his last birthday. I remember suddenly being unable to see what I was writing on the card for tears, but that wasn't the prevailing mood because Aron decided to celebrate. There were quite a lot of birthday cards, and one had champagne bottles on it. Aron said he would like champagne. He would like a party. Danny and his wife and child were to be invited to come over.

Danny's wife Rachel's pregnancy at that time made her

127

even more sweet and placid than usual. Aron and she used to get on very well together, but everybody got on well with her. She was so good at listening to other people. However, the party didn't quite work out as planned. Aron had really withdrawn too far from the outside world by now. I wasn't surprised when he decided not to have the whole company in his room. Several people there at the same time would in itself have been so shattering a change. In the end, the party took place downstairs. Only Danny and I moved from one room to the other. But Aron was still determined to celebrate.

'How would it be if I took champagne?' he asked Danny.

'I think it would do you good. I think you'd enjoy it.'

Aron tried some, sitting propped up against his pillows.

'Yes,' he said, smiling and slipping down the bed a little. 'Yes, it's good!'

After a few more thimblefuls he became quite gay. Or rather, the underlying gaiety that seemed to me characteristic of him at that time, came to the surface. We all began to laugh. I suppose a few thimblefuls of champagne affected me fairly strongly too. I remember feeling how fundamentally, deeply right our laughter was. There was unaccountable contentment everywhere. For a short time after that, Aron and I used to drink small quantities of champagne together quite often.

Meanwhile the enemy made new inroads. One morning Aron woke up to find his left arm so weak that he was incapable of raising it. He had virtually lost the use of it. He seemed unsurprised. We both behaved as if this were the sort of thing that happens every day. But I was very sad about that arm. Nothing that went wrong with Aron's body was likely ever to be righted now. I grieved over each new injury that the disease inflicted on something that had been so beautiful and young and strong.

I cherished what was left. I seemed at times to be enormously busy just doing what there was to keep his body comfortable: rubbing his back and heels with surgical spirit, re-making the bed, adjusting the pillows, renewing the mouthwash. Danny offered many suggestions for relief and comfort. On his advice we bought a large piece of foam rubber for Aron to lie on. I cut a hole in this where the bone at the base of his spine protruded—the spot where the pressure was most likely to result in a bedsore.

The day his arm went wrong, it was difficult to change his pyjama jacket. He was listening to the record from the soundtrack of *Jules et Jim* at the time.

'Happy days!' he said, as he rolled on to his side to let me put the weak arm into its sleeve. I had to blank out *Jules et Jim* from my mind. To look back was impossible.

This was the day after Dr. Sidebotham's regular weekly visit, and there seemed no point in trying to call him in specially about Aron's arm. To boost our morale, Danny took a constructive line. He suggested that the debility was due to a deficiency of a certain vitamin, and that injections of this might help. I doubt if anybody actually believed that these injections would cure Aron's arm, but Aron himself was keen on trying them.

This was what Dr. Sidebotham called 'clutching at straws'. He could never understand this attitude. When he paid his next visit, he took as serious a view of the arm as I knew he would. I suppose that this was really why I had been in no hurry to tell him about it. He diagnosed it as the result of secondary deposits on the right side of the brain, and stepped up his visits to twice weekly after that. Also, either then or shortly afterwards, he told my parents that it would be wiser to stop Aron from walking to the bathroom. His heart might not be able to stand the strain. My parents said no. They said that if Aron and I thought this possible, we shouldn't be discouraged. In fact, Aron went on getting up until practically the end.

Perhaps Dr. Sidebotham was right about Aron's arm, but I never accepted this diagnosis. I never saw any evidence that there was anything wrong with Aron's brain. But the doctor's opposition to the vitamin injections was certainly well-intentioned. He was genuinely sorry to think of Aron getting any more injections than he actually needed. He thought it cruelty. You needed to be very close to Aron to know how very little a few more pinpricks bothered him.

'Would you give him one of these injections yourself?' he asked me.

Missing the point and assuming that he spoke of injections in general, I explained that my mother had offered to do this.

'But, yes,' I said. 'If it depended on me I would.'

Dr. Sidebotham sadly relented, prescribed the vitamin and gave the first injection himself. He implied, however, that he would prefer it if somebody else continued this particular treatment. Mrs. Polly did so with enthusiasm. She said the vitamin had done many of her patients a great deal of good. She believed in it absolutely.

I was glad to see Aron getting anything that might conceivably be therapeutic. I wished he could have food injected. I thought that we should all be putting up the maximum possible fight, because that's what Aron was doing himself.

> 'Do not go gentle into that good night.
> Rage, rage against the dying of the light.'

Strange things have happened. Even cancer has been known to recede and disappear. Sometimes I thought that Aron might have lived longer had I been strong enough to refute the medical evidence from the outset. Mr. Warfield-Scrogge had really succeeded only too well in convincing me that Aron was going to die. Consequently there were always limits to my idea of what the maximum possible fight was. I never tried to persuade Aron to go downstairs, for instance. Yet he might have done it, had I behaved as if I thought it possible. Probably it wasn't possible. But who knows? Anything was worth trying. Only resignation was wrong.

Aron had enormous inner resources. Nothing seemed to affect the core of him at all. He was still capable, for example, of getting up for most of an afternoon and writing as many as ten or twelve letters to record companies and jazz magazines. He was still using a remarkable amount of this time as if it were a holiday, a chance to think and listen to music and catch up on his reading. In fact, he went on adding to the list of books he'd read until the day before he died. Then it just stopped, the handwriting as clear and strong as ever, as if some sudden unexpected accident and not a slow malignancy had cut him off. What he read then was equally incredible. It embraced so much: Aristophanes and Christopher Fry, Dickens and Evelyn Waugh, H. G. Wells and Edmund Gosse, practically all the anthologies of poetry in the flat.

My very few excursions to the outside world were to the local library to borrow records for him—plays as well as music. I remember him simultaneously reading and listening to *A Midsummer Night's Dream*, with no apparent loss of concentration from the old days. His mind seemed independent of the illness. He could describe even his own condition almost dispassionately now.

'I want to eat,' he once said, 'but the trouble is I can't absorb the food.'

Nonetheless he kept trying to digest enough to stay alive. He tried anything that there was any hope of keeping down: meat drinks and soups and complan, which he disliked however it was flavoured. He drank large quantities of Vichy water in the hope that it would do him good.

Although the morphia injections were an immense relief, he regarded them in the same way as the pills. He tried to have as few as possible. He never had them at fixed times, and sometimes he had very few indeed. He had them at irregular intervals to mitigate the chaotic feeling that, as time went on, became less easy to describe as simply pain. As far as I could tell, he was never reliant on morphia, never addicted.

In fact, he refused to give in on any front. He wanted life more the harder it became. And it was very hard now. His mouth was all furred up and sore. On Dr. Sidebotham's advice he used to suck fresh pineapple or tinned pineapple cubes in an attempt to counteract this. His legs were swollen with oedema, so that any finger-tip pressure on them made an indentation that remained there. His stomach was swollen too. I thought of this, perhaps wrongly, as the cancer itself. He usually got up for shorter times now, and occasionally didn't want to move at all. It was becoming increasingly difficult to rub his back enough, and there was a red patch developing on the point that took most of the pressure. Sometimes his whole body was so tormented that the weight of even a blanket was more than he could bear. He would say this was because he was too hot. He never described any of these things as painful. But even to him, they must have added up to a sense of total discomfort.

Until then I would have been terrified to confront a human being in such a condition. But this was Aron, and so the condition was only part of what I saw. Actually, I have difficulty now in conjuring up an accurate picture of him then. I grasped the details, but never really saw the whole thing as others did. What I remember clearly is beautiful: Aron like a wild, emaciated poet with his huge eyes and red-gold hair grown long, suddenly picking up a vase of sweet-scented freesia and burying his face in it. His eyes, I think, are what I remember best—the love that was always in them.

By the end, nobody else could begin to fill the gap created by my absence from his bedside. He needed me most after dark. Once I left him in the late evening, to have a bath. I was away too long. I know what happened. All round him there was emptiness, a horrid void into which pieces of him were falling, slipping, sliding away beyond the point where anything could bank them up. Finally in desperation, he startled us all by knocking on the floor with a stick that we had given him for this purpose but which he almost never used. I rushed back quickly to stop his whole world from disintegrating.

Christmas was coming, and cards started to arrive. I was relieved to see them because I'd had an irrational fear that some of our silent friends might behave as if Aron was already dead. Aron showed considerable interest in the cards, and insisted that everybody who sent one should get one back.

'On Christmas day,' he said happily, 'you must all come into my room, all of you.'

Perhaps he was going to make Christmas after all. I thought it a pity that Mr. Warfield-Scrogge was unaware of what was going on. How would he react to a Christmas card from Aron and me? I didn't send one, of course, but there was a buoyancy about my attitude then that seems, in retrospect, extraordinary, out of all relation to the grimness of the facts.

Mrs. Polly was having a holiday at Christmas. Other nurses would temporarily take over from her. It was a pity, but it couldn't be helped. We gave her a small present, and exchanged Christmas greetings before she left.

'I do hope he will be able to enjoy it a little,' she said to my mother and me on the way out. 'He is so nice, such a nice person, and so cheerful.'

'I wonder what she was thinking,' I remarked as we watched her pedalling up the street.

'I think she expects to find us all here after Christmas, if that's what you mean,' my mother said.

I didn't think so. I had the feeling that she expected never to see Aron again.

Mrs. Polly's temporary replacement was a Mrs. Smith, a very loquacious woman who rarely seemed to give her patient the whole of her attention. She talked about things like house prices, waving her hands in the air, while Aron lay in a painful position waiting for her to finish what she was doing. He had a bedsore now that all our efforts had failed to prevent and it needed daily dressing.

Not surprisingly perhaps, Mrs. Smith was also bureaucratic. Many nurses join the domiciliary services in order to escape this feature of the hospital regime, but she wasn't one. She insisted on introducing a correct system for everything, regardless of the efficiency of the system already operating. She objected, for instance, to ampoules of morphia lying anywhere in sight, as if the room were a public place where any passer-by might give himself a fix. Once she tidied away the box of syringes so

133

effectively that I couldn't find it when it was next needed. There was quite a panic until it was discovered, well concealed from us, but plainly visible to the outside world, behind the curtains on the window sill.

I was rather concerned that this nurse should not be the one who was around when things got really serious. She represented too much of what we had succeeded in escaping. Fortunately there was another, very young nurse, who paid some visits at this point, and whose telephone number we had. This Miss Martin was exceptionally willing, and in fact told us to feel free to phone her at any time.

'Do you really mean *any* time?' I asked.

'Of course.'

'What about Christmas?'

'Just ring me and I'll come. Even if I'm eating my Christmas dinner, I'll come.'

12

It was the day before Christmas Eve. I had been lying awake for some time before I got up, put on my dressing gown and opened the curtains a little. A solitary seagull floated across the leaden winter sky. It was a long way from the sea for the bird to have come.

Aron was still asleep. He hadn't stirred even when I let in the light. It had been 1 a.m. before we settled the previous night; Aron was at the same time very tired and very restless, like somebody who had been shut indoors for far too long. He had finally asked for an injection although he said he wasn't actually in pain. It seemed like a kind of desperate measure to counteract something he couldn't describe and couldn't name, and my mother was sad about giving the injection.

It was nearly nine now. However long it took him to go to sleep Aron was usually wide awake by then. I went and stood beside his bed.

'Aron, are you awake?' I said very quietly.

His eyes opened wide. He blinked. He was miles and miles away. I could see him struggling to come nearer. It took him a full minute to reach the surface. When he finally spoke his voice was thick with sleep—or something worse. He looked a little startled and yet happy, happy to have dragged himself back to me, happy to be facing another day. We both smiled.

A few minutes later I went downstairs and looked out of the window to see if Danny's car was still in the street.

'I think we'd better ask Danny to look in, if he can,' I said to my mother.

'Is Aron worse then?' she asked sadly. She had grown enormously attached to the gentle, uncomplaining invalid, around whom she made the household revolve.

'He took a terribly long time to waken up.'

My voice was flat and empty. I knew very well that the battle couldn't last much longer. I dreaded the coma that the sister had predicted. I dreaded the moment when he became inaccessible to me, my love, my comfort.

My mother went and spoke to Danny, who came to see Aron very soon after. He must have formed an impression similar to mine, for he told me that he would be around all day, and said to call him if I felt at all worried. He added that he would come back later in any case to see how we were getting on. He advised me meanwhile not to do anything at all, just to let Aron rest.

Aron had no desire to do anything that day, not even to read or listen to music. He just lay there watching while I strung Christmas cards along the wall. Then I sat holding his hand. A great quietness descended on the room.

At some point in the morning he began to sweat profusely. I put a towel under his hands because the sheet was becoming so wet. Danny, who was on the scene again already, suggested giving him an aspirin to try to bring his temperature down. Aron swallowed the aspirin dissolved in water, although he hadn't been able to bring himself to eat or drink anything else that day. It was incredible what he could still force himself to do if it was likely to improve his condition. Obviously he was fighting, as best he could, still.

Outside the door of the room, I told Danny how concerned I was about the small amount of nourishment that Aron had had in the past few days. I was afraid that if he didn't eat more, he would die because of that. Danny told me not to worry. It was surprising, he said, how long people could survive without food. He told me on no account to agitate Aron in any way.

136

At this point Mrs. Smith appeared, but to my relief Danny told her that there was nothing she could do at present. He asked her, however, to come back in the late afternoon.

It was a strange day, all still and heavy like the weather. Minute by minute, the life I loved was ticking away, and there was absolutely nothing to be done about it.

Suddenly, in the afternoon, Aron tried to rouse himself.

'Why am I in this state?' he said.

'Because you're ill.' I mopped his brow.

'What does Danny say?'

'He says you'll probably want to rest most of the day.'

A little later Aron decided to try to drink some orange juice. Swallowing it made him start coughing. It was an awful cough, a cough that caught at his breathing and tore his whole body. He rolled painfully on to his side in an attempt to get some air.

'I think I'd better get Danny,' I said, because Aron had never been like this before.

'No . . .' Aron caught at my hand. He thought I was going to leave him.

'I won't go away,' I said quickly. 'I won't leave you. I'll just knock.'

I banged on the floor with Aron's stick, and my mother appeared at once. I asked her to get Danny. I insisted that she should phone him and not go out of the flat. It was such an illogical thing to be insisting on at this moment, so unimportant and irrelevant, that it must have had some deeper significance. My father had to stay in too. In my mind perhaps we were consolidating our forces against an unseen invader, closing the ranks of love and affection—something like that.

Danny was almost immediately in the room.

'Aron tried to drink some orange juice,' I said.

Aron's breathing was now very loud and heavy, as if the orange juice had stuck in his lungs. Danny very gently tapped his back.

'He hasn't actually got a pain,' I said. 'But he's feeling pretty bad. Do you think an injection would help?'

Aron hadn't had any drugs, other than the aspirin, all day, and I thought morphia might make him feel better. It was the only thing there was to do.

'Do you want me to give you an injection?' Danny asked Aron. He never gave an injection without saying this first.

'Yes please,' Aron said.

Danny gave the injection. Then I sat down in my usual position close beside Aron, and Danny took a chair at the other side of the room.

After a little Aron smiled and said he felt much better now. But his voice was thick and difficult to make out.

'What next?' he asked, looking quite confident that whatever it was would be pleasant.

'The nurse will probably come back soon,' Danny said. 'We'll give her ten minutes, and if she doesn't come we'll change your bed to make you more comfortable.'

'Fine,' said Aron. He had been sweating so much that all his bed linen was soaking.

'Please don't let the nurse come,' I willed silently.

She didn't come, and Danny and I started to change Aron's things. There was only a faint scar now, where the huge wound from the operation had been. It seemed incredible that none of this colossal healing power could have been harnessed to fight the cancer.

I was standing at the bottom of the bed when Aron said, 'I can't see you properly.' I moved right up beside him, and kissed his forehead.

'Can you see me now?'

'Yes.'

I sat there for a moment, holding him. Then imagining the crisis to be over, I got up and started to fold a sheet lengthwise with Danny.

Aron's eyes followed me round the bed. He was smiling. I gave a little laugh because his expression was so pleasant. And then I stopped in my tracks. Danny seemed to be thinking there was something wrong. He was examining Aron closely, listening to his heart. He pulled the clean sheet across Aron's shoulder.

'I think he's passed on,' he said.

'He means dead,' I thought, 'dead'. But I just stood there looking at Aron's smiling face. It was a strange elusive smile, impossible to interpret, hard to be sure of even.

'Do you think so?' I said at last.

'Yes.'

'He's smiling, isn't he?'

'Yes.'

A long moment passed. Then Danny said, 'I'll leave you for a minute.' And he went out of the room.

I moved my chair close up to Aron, and clung to him, and suddenly started to sob and cry.

Yet when Danny reappeared, and for a long time afterwards, I kept reiterating, 'Are you sure?' Aron's hands were warm. He still looked the same. I kept suggesting that he might not, after all, be dead.

It seemed like several hours before I could be persuaded to walk out of that room. When I did, I was conscious of my hands dangling uselessly by my sides. I was a person with no job to do, no place to fill, no function in life. The line had been drawn—the line between the world that contained somebody who needed me, and the world that had to go on somehow without him.

*　　*　　*

In the living room my parents welcomed me almost as if I had come back from the dead. They did their utmost, at that moment, to show there were still people to whom my existence mattered.

My father and Danny had already been busy making arrangements for the funeral. I had said that they should do whatever they thought best. It didn't seem to matter greatly, once Aron was dead, what happened to what remained of him. His parents wanted him to be cremated and I wanted that too, because his body had had enough.

Then it became apparent that if the present plans went forward, the undertakers would be coming shortly to take his body away to a Chapel of Rest. That did matter. I felt he had to have a funeral from his own home, not somewhere anonymous where he had never been and never would have gone. Even the name 'Chapel of Rest' seemed to me so euphemistic, such a pretence. It was death, not rest, that we were dealing with, and somehow it wasn't over yet. There still remained some need to see it through—for me, I think, not for Aron now. His death was part of my life, and I needed time to look at it and understand that it had really happened.

My parents agreed at once about this.

'Sending him away then would have been almost as bad as letting him go back to hospital,' my mother remarked afterwards. They rang the undertakers, and arranged that the body would remain at home until the cremation. Someone would call at the flat the following day to do whatever embalming was necessary. There was difficulty, however, in fixing the cremation date anywhere in the near future at all. Perhaps, if the body is in a Chapel of Rest, people don't mind waiting longer. It was then the day before Christmas Eve, a Thursday. Friday was too soon. Saturday was Christmas Day. Sunday was out. Monday was another holiday. Tuesday was heavily booked up. The undertakers suggested Wednesday.

'But that's nearly a week!' I exclaimed. 'That's far too long!'

I suddenly found myself holding the phone and arguing with the undertakers. I would certainly have claimed at the same time that there was nothing left to fight for any more, but fighting becomes a sort of habit I suppose.

The thing was finally fixed up for Tuesday at a different crematorium from the one originally planned. We had five nights and practically five days now just to wait until it was all over. Christmas Day would be the worst, I thought, the day that Aron had wanted us all to come to his room. I would have given anything to have been able to exchange just one more sentence, one more glance with him. 'If two people love each other there can be no happy end to it.' Aron had noted down the quotation from Hemingway long before any of this began to happen.

The studio couch on which I slept was moved downstairs into the living room. There was nothing to hope for now except that the body wouldn't alter too much before his parents saw it on the day of the cremation. Perhaps even the smile might stay to give them a kind of peace. I wanted the embalmer to come quickly.

But before the embalmer came, there was a succession of events that would certainly have appealed to Aron's sense of the farcical. The number of doctors who called at the house, for instance, now there was nothing helpful any of them could do, would have amazed and delighted him. Although he had, in the opinion of the medical profession, been at the point of death for over two months, it seemed to be quite a tricky business to prove that he had actually died. Bureaucracy pursued him still.

Danny, it emerged, was ineligible to sign the certificate, I think because he qualified in another country and hadn't yet been long enough on the British register. So a doctor whom none of us had ever seen before was called in to sign the thing and receive the two guinea fee.

Then some hitch necessitated a repeat performance of the signing of the certificate the next morning. Practically the first sight that greeted us after we got up on Christmas Eve was this great gathering of doctors round the breakfast table— Dr. Sidebotham, the strange doctor and Danny, all hard at it filling in the document again. The document itself was essential. The embalmer couldn't touch the body until the local Registrar had issued a death certificate in exchange for it. The Registrar was available only at certain rather restricted times, and it became something of a rush to ensure that the embalmer would be able to come at all that day. It couldn't have been done without a car and several people willing to co-operate.

The embalmer was gentle and sympathetic. He seemed to care about Aron, or what death had left of him. But somehow, when he had finished his work, there was only an empty shell where Aron had been.

'Aron's not there,' I said. The smile, the expression, everything had gone. Where was he then? Where had he gone? Because if he wasn't in that body, he must be somewhere. Religion could have provided such consoling answers.

A strange thing was that for quite a long time afterwards, I felt as if something of him carried on in me. I felt as if I resembled him in the occasional expression, gesture, mannerism. But I think this was never noticeable to anybody else.

I was reluctant to leave the flat until after the cremation, and most of the time we just sat around. And sometimes visitors came. After dark on Christmas Eve, during a heavy rainstorm, the doorbell rang. My mother went to answer it. Standing there in the rain was a woman of some presence whom she had never met. She waited for the stranger to speak.

'Dr. Sciberas,' the other introduced herself.

'O-oh!' my mother was astonished.

'How is Mrs. Evans?' the doctor asked.

'Not particularly well,' my mother said.

'Would she like to see me?'

'I doubt it but I'll ask her.'

My mother left the doctor at the door and came into the living room.

'Do you want to see Dr. Sciberas?' she said to me.

'No,' I replied.

'No,' my mother told the doctor, who turned on her heel and left.

I think it amazed us all that now, when nobody needed her, Dr. Sciberas had finally chosen to come. I would get another doctor later I supposed. Meanwhile there was nothing that Dr. Sciberas and I could possibly talk about. The struggle, in which she hadn't wanted to be involved, was still the only thing that mattered to me. It was what kept me going for ages afterwards, the triumph of knowing that Aron and I had never given in.

*   *   *

It was a beautiful day, the day of the cremation. The sun made the frost sparkle and the sky was suffused with gold. Lots of our friends came and there were flowers everywhere—so many reasons for having done his utmost not to die.

I agreed to a short service at the crematorium. Some ceremony was needed, and this was what our parents wanted. I had no reason really to revolt in public against a Presbyterian childhood that had given me such a sound basis for future independence. Aron had always hated public exhibitions of any kind. And perhaps the others got some comfort from the minister's suggestion that this death was, in a way, a merciful release.

Date Due

78